THE
CARBOHYDRATE ADDICT'S
NO CRAVINGS
COOKBOOK

200 All-New Low-Carb Recipes
to Satisfy Every Craving

OTHER BOOKS BY DRS. RACHAEL AND RICHARD HELLER

The Carbohydrate Addict's 7-Day Plan

The Carbohydrate Addict's LifeSpan Program

The Carbohydrate Addict's Carbohydrate Counter

The Carbohydrate Addict's Fat Counter

The Carbohydrate Addict's Calorie Counter

The Carbohydrate Addict's Gram Counter

The Carbohydrate Addict's Diet

The Carbohydrate Addict's Program for Success

The Carbohydrate Addict's Cookbook

The Carbohydrate Addict's Healthy Heart Program

The Carbohydrate Addict's Healthy for Life Plan

Carbohydrate-Addicted Kids

THE
CARBOHYDRATE ADDICT'S NO CRAVINGS COOKBOOK

200 All-New Low-Carb Recipes
to Satisfy Every Craving

Rachael F. Heller, M.A., M.Ph., Ph.D.

Assistant Clinical Professor, Mount Sinai School of Medicine, New York;
Assistant Professor, Graduate Center of the City University of New York,
Department of Biomedical Sciences, retired

Richard F. Heller, M.S., Ph.D.

Professor, Mount Sinai School of Medicine, New York, retired;
Professor, Graduate Center of the City University of New York,
Department of Biomedical Sciences, retired;
Professor Emeritus, City University of New York

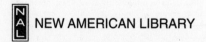 NEW AMERICAN LIBRARY

New American Library
Published by New American Library, a division of Penguin Group (USA) Inc., 375 Hudson Street,
New York, New York 10014, USA
Penguin Group (Canada), 90 Eglinton Avenue East, Suite 700, Toronto,
Ontario M4P 2Y3, Canada (a division of Pearson Penguin Canada Inc.)
Penguin Books Ltd., 80 Strand, London WC2R 0RL, England
Penguin Ireland, 25 St. Stephen's Green, Dublin 2,
Ireland (a division of Penguin Books Ltd.)
Penguin Group (Australia), 250 Camberwell Road, Camberwell, Victoria 3124,
Australia (a division of Pearson Australia Group Pty. Ltd.)
Penguin Books India Pvt. Ltd., 11 Community Centre, Panchsheel Park,
New Delhi - 110 017, India
Penguin Group (NZ), cnr Airborne and Rosedale Roads, Albany,
Auckland 1310, New Zealand (a division of Pearson New Zealand Ltd.)
Penguin Books (South Africa) (Pty.) Ltd., 24 Sturdee Avenue,
Rosebank, Johannesburg 2196, South Africa

Penguin Books Ltd., Registered Offices:
80 Strand, London WC2R 0RL, England

Published by New American Library, a division of Penguin Group (USA) Inc. Previously published in a
Dutton edition.

First New American Library Printing, January 2006
10 9 8 7 6 5 4 3 2 1

 REGISTERED TRADEMARK—MARCA REGISTRADA

New American Library Trade Paperback ISBN: 0-451-21743-8

The Library of Congress has cataloged the hardcover edition of this title as follows:

Heller, Rachael F.
The carbohydrate addict's no cravings cookbook : 200 all-new low-carb recipes to satisfy every craving /
Rachael F. Heller, Richard F. Heller.
p cm.
ISBN 0-525-948554-4
1. Low-carbohydrate diet—Recipes.   I. Heller, Richard F.   II. Title.
RM237.73.H452 2004
641.5'6383—dc22   2004058238

Set in Sabon
Designed by Leonard Telesca

Printed in the United States of America

To all of us who refuse to give up pleasure
in order to be happy

CONTENTS

ACKNOWLEDGMENTS

We wish to express our deep appreciation to:

Mel Berger, Senior Vice President, William Morris Agency. His thoughtful and incisive advice, exceptional mind, creativity, commitment, and vision make him the best agent in the world. In addition, his insight and brilliant sense of humor never fail to amaze us.

Carole Baron, President of Dutton, whose well-respected experience, thought, and energy have been invaluable.

Kara Welsh, Publisher, New American Library, and Brian Tart, Publisher, Dutton Books, for their unswerving commitment to excellence in publishing and to bringing to low-carb dieters—without delay—the information they need to separate the real from the hype.

Liz Perl, Vice President and Director of Marketing, New American Library, our beloved publicist, who has worked tirelessly and intelligently on so many of our projects, getting vital information to those who needed it when they needed it. A joy to know and work with as well, her energy, fine professional judgment, and unswerving commitment make her one in a trillion.

Ellen Edwards, Executive Editor, New American Library, our wonderful editor, for her relentless work under pressure, untiring interest, concern, commitment, and willingness to go the extra mile (time and time again) to get the job done (and done with excellence). Beyond all she does every day, for her brilliant editing.

Susan Schwartz, Managing Editor of Dutton, our production and design fairy godmother who gets it all together and makes it all work—beautifully.

Anthony Ramondo, Art Director, New American Library, who takes old photos and partial ideas, sprinkles them with imagination, creativity, and pixie dust, and makes magic.

Eric Lupfer, Mel Berger's most capable and intelligent assistant, for his trusted reliability and unflagging involvement.

Craig Burke, Director of Publicity, New American Library, whose excellence and hard work is greatly appreciated.

Heather Connor, Publicist, New American Library, our affable, tireless, and brilliant liaison to the media and the world.

Serena Jones, Editorial Assistant to Ellen Edwards, for her continued attention and tireless help (even while being challenged with a world of other demands).

Liz Perl's wonderful staff of publicists and marketing assistants at New American Library, who are always there when we need them most to do the work they do so well.

Rob Schloss and his exceptional assistants, Michele Martin and Chelsea Bauman, for their interest, daily input, critical advice, and well-considered suggestions.

Nick D'Amato and Casmera Grove, our most excellent computer and technical advisors, who each manage to combine brilliance with a caring and loving spirit. Their concern (when no one else cared) and help (when no one else could have helped) have saved our necks and our work, as well. Their forward vision and talent never cease to amaze us.

The Apple Computer Company and their support staff, for the development, care, and "feeding" of our user-friendly Macintosh laptops and desktops, which have made our lives a joy and have been invaluable tools in all of our work. Apple's excellent repair team keeps us up and running, and Apple's patient support staff regularly leads us out of the dark tech forest into the light. Apple's hard work and high standards have made our work both easy and productive. Because of Apple, we're proud to say, we don't do windows.

INTRODUCTION

JUST FOR YOU

This cookbook was created for your pleasure—and your pleasure alone.

In the pages that follow you will *not* find recipes to delight your friends, excite your family, or entertain your guests. There are no tips on preparing large family dinners or holiday parties. Instead, the dishes here have been developed to please your taste buds, cater to your needs, and satisfy your cravings so that you can stay on your low-carb eating program without sacrifice or deprivation.

We have *not* divided this book into neat sections devoted to breakfast, lunch, and dinner. Instead, the recipes have been organized around specific cravings—so that you can find the kind of food you want when you want it. It's the craving you seek to satisfy, not the time of day.

If Richard and I had our way, each recipe would have a serving size of one, maybe two. It is a point of fact, however, that combining ingredients, especially in low-carb cooking, doesn't work that way. Most dishes need a minimum of two to four servings to achieve an ideal balance of flavors. Although a dish may provide multiple servings, they are all *yours* to enjoy. Refrigerate them for a day or two, warm them up or enjoy them cold, or freeze them for the next time a craving hits.

So leave behind the needs and desires of the rest of the world and get ready to focus on meeting *your* weight-loss goals and satisfying *your* cravings. Chances are, you're long overdue for some well-deserved rewards of your own.

HEALTHY SELFISHNESS

You've planned and shopped and cooked for others. You've sliced, diced, and sautéed until you were blue in the face. You've scrubbed the pots and taken care of the dishes and, if you were lucky, very lucky, you've heard the words "This is good," mumbled through a food-packed mouth or two. And you've wondered when you were going to break free of the endless chore of taking care of other people.

Well, welcome to a little bit of healthy selfishness, where what *you* want counts—your dreams for tomorrow *and* your desires for today—a haven where you can lose weight without deprivation and indulge your cravings without guilt.

Most of all, healthy selfishness is learning to listen to the little voice inside of you that has been told to be quiet for too long, that has started speaking in barely perceptible whispers, and that longs to shout to the world, "This is my life, too!"

For us, personally, that voice has been our savior. Once we learned to honor it and stand up for it, we were able to lose a combined two hundred pounds and keep the weight off, without deprivation, for more than two decades.

You have heard the experts attest to the fact that weight loss requires extraordinary discipline and sacrifice. Our answer: Bull! Self-sacrificing feats of restraint and abstinence can work for only so long. In the end, the human need for comfort and pleasure almost inevitably wins out.

A successful weight-loss program requires, most of all, a commitment to treat yourself well, to put your own needs first, and to fully enjoy the pleasure that food was meant to provide.

Chances are you've tried the sacrifice approach . . . many times. It simply doesn't work. Now it's time to listen to that little voice inside you and indulge in a bit of well-earned healthy selfishness.

It works. We know and we have proof; actually more than two hundred pounds' worth!

PLANNING FOR PLEASURE

If you were to have guests for dinner—family, friends, even strangers—chances are you would plan your meal in advance. You'd choose the recipes, buy the food, and prepare the dishes after carefully considering all your options. Isn't it odd, then, that most low-carb dieters rarely plan their own meals ahead of time—giving little or no thought to the new and exciting dishes with which they might please themselves?

As a first step toward incorporating a bit of healthy selfishness in your life, we encourage you to plan for pleasure. Take the same time, energy, and interest that you would give to your family, friends, kids, a family pet, even a perfect stranger, and think about what *you* would like to eat. Choose the recipes you want to enjoy, purchase the ingredients you need on hand to make them, and take the time to prepare the low-carb dishes that best suit your diet. Go ahead and cook up a storm—with just your needs and desires in mind. You'll find it's time well spent.

A SIMPLE GUIDE TO CARB COUNTS AND INGREDIENTS

In the recipes that follow, carb counts are always given in total carb grams per serving. All carb counts are rounded to the nearest whole number. If a serving contains less than one-half gram of carbohydrates per serving, it is rounded to 0 (zero). If it contains more than one-half gram but less than one gram of carbohydrates per serving, it is rounded to 1 (one).

Unless otherwise indicated, the size of vegetables or other ingredients is considered to be "average" and carb counts are calculated in the same way.

Where onions, cabbage, or other ingredients are not specified by variety, the choice is yours. You may prefer the less pungent taste of a white onion instead of a yellow one, for instance, or your supermarket may generally carry only one or two varieties of cabbage. Unless indicated, we have found the specific variety makes little difference to either the taste or the carb count.

The recipes list ingredients simply as "sour cream" or "sausage" or "bacon," etc. At the supermarket, however, you will face a myriad of choices: ten types of sour cream (low-fat, low-carb, all natural, etc.) and a dozen different sausages and bacons (sugar-free, low-salt, organic, etc.). For these and other ingredients, the variety (and the pros and cons of each choice) can present an almost overwhelming dilemma. Choose "low-fat" and you may be getting an item higher in carbs. Choose "sugar-free" and the product may include a hefty portion of sugar substitutes. Choose something that claims to be "low-carb" and you may not really be getting low-carb at all.

Our recommendation is, as always, to consult with your physician to determine your weight-loss and health priorities. If low-carb is your only goal, then avoid any prepared food in our recipes that contains sugar as an ingredient. (Almost any ingredient ending in "-ose" as well as a variety of corn syrups are names for sugars.) If saturated fats are also of concern, learn the names of the fats you should avoid and, again, pay attention to the ingredient list and nutrition label. And so on.

You'll see that we've listed olive oil as the preferred cooking oil. In doing so, we considered the levels of saturated fats in a variety of oils as well as the level of monounsaturated fats, the smoking points, and the amount of omega-3 versus omega-6, both desirable oils. Since omega-3 is found in meats, fish, and vegetables, and is more likely to be consumed already by low-carb dieters, we thought it best to recommend an oil high in omega-6, that is, olive oil. In addition, for each recipe we chose the oil whose flavor best suits the other ingredients. As always, however, the needs of your particular eating program, as determined by you and your physician, should prevail. If your physician recommends canola oil rather than olive oil, for example, that recommendation should supersede our ingredients list.

While all of the recipes is this book are low in carbohydrates (not just in net carbs but in total carbs), some may be more in keeping with your personal health-related goals. Enjoy on a regular basis those recipes that best fit all of your needs, and save others for special occasions. Even better, be creative and replace less-preferable ingredients with those that better meet your personal requirements. Feel free to substitute bacon with chicken or fish, for example, or enjoy a low-fat cheese rather than a higher-fat variety.

This is your cookbook as well as your life. The choices you make can help you rewrite both.

GLUTAMATES: UNWANTED ADDITIONS

Glutamates, including but not limited to MSG (monosodium glutamate), are chemicals in food that are found naturally or, in the case of processed food, are added. When glutamates occur naturally, they don't seem to cause significant problems for most dieters. When glutamates are added to processed foods, however, they can lead to increased hunger, cravings, and weight gain. Some individuals are quite sensitive to added glutamates, while others are not.

Food manufacturers add glutamates to food to make it taste better and to keep the consumer coming back to buy more. Glutamates may be present in foods under any of the following names (found in the products' ingredient list):

anything enzyme modified
anything fermented
anything protein fortified
anything ultra pasteurized
autolyzed yeast
barley malt
broth
bouillon
calcium caseinate
carrageen
flavoring
gelatin
hydrolyzed oat flour
hydrolyzed plant protein
hydrolyzed vegetable protein
hydrolyzed soy protein
malt extract
maltodextrin
natural flavor(ing)
pectin
plant protein extract
potassium glutamate
sodium caseinate
soy protein
soy sauce
stock
textured protein
whey protein
yeast extract
yeast food

As a low-carb dieter, you might find it helpful to avoid processed condiments such as hot sauce, mayonnaise, and prepared horseradish that contain these additives. You might even decide you want to make your own condiments. We've included three recipes for homemade hot sauce, beginning on page 259, to get you started.

If you find yourself unexplainably drawn to a certain brand of food, you may want to check its ingredient list for any of the above items. We advise you to check with your physician if you have uncontrollable cravings for any food.

For more information on glutamates and their effects on your insulin levels, hunger, cravings, weight gain, and the ability to stay on a weight-loss program, see our *Carbohydrate Addict's 7-Day Plan* or *The Carbohydrate Addict's LifeSpan Program.*

AN EASY BUT ESSENTIAL TOFU TIP

One of the many delights of cooking with tofu is that it takes on the flavors of all of the herbs and spices with which it is cooked—but only if it is drained of the excess liquid in which it is packed.

We have discovered a simple and quick technique for draining the excess liquid from the tofu block without damaging the tofu so that, like a rich sponge, it can soak up the wonderful flavors of the dish you are preparing:

To get your tofu ready for cooking, lay the block on its larger side on a clean, dry dinner plate. Gently stack three dinner plates on top of the block, in an even distribution of weight. The weight will exert a slow pressure on the tofu and liquid will begin to pool at the base of tofu in the plate.

Place the tofu and plates in the refrigerator for 1 hour, returning every 10 to 15 minutes to check for and drain the pooled liquid.

After one hour, remove the tofu from the refrigerator, drain the last pool of liquid, and use the tofu as directed in the recipe.

ONE LAST THOUGHT

Each recipe in the pages that follow is low enough in carbs to comply with virtually any low-carb diet. Rather than being faced with cumbersome carb counting, your challenge will be this: to answer the question, "What am I craving right now?"

With that answer in mind, or with a desire just to browse, look over the fifteen sections in the Contents (page ix), listed by cravings. From "Chinese Delights" to "Italian Indulgences," from "Crunchy Satisfaction" to "Comfort Food," each section in this book will provide you with at least thirteen low-carb choices (a baker's dozen) to make you feel good all over.

WHAT ARE YOU CRAVING?

BARBECUE BOUNTY

Cajun Grill

PREP TIME: 5 minutes

COOK TIME: 1 hour

SERVINGS: 4

CARBS PER SERVING: 2 grams

When nothing but the tangy taste of barbecue will do, this quick fix works wonders. The dish that inspired our version was served to us in a tiny bed-and-breakfast in New Orleans where Sue and Alan, the owners, threw a cookout in our honor. They had lost a combined forty pounds eating low-carb and wanted to show us that they could cook Cajun without the carbohydrates.

1   cup white vinegar
2   teaspoons paprika (hot or sweet)
2   teaspoons Dijon mustard
1   tablespoon dried basil

1/2   teaspoon cayenne pepper (or as desired)
1   cup olive oil
Salt and pepper, as desired
1 1/2   pounds chicken legs, backs, quarters, or wings

In a medium-size bowl, combine the vinegar, paprika, mustard, basil, cayenne pepper, olive oil, and salt and pepper as desired, to form a marinade. Mix well.

Add the raw chicken and stir so that all the surfaces of the chicken are exposed to the marinade. Cover the bowl and place it in the refrigerator for 1 hour.

Remove the chicken from the refrigerator and discard the marinade before cooking. Do *not* use the marinade for basting. Either grill the chicken on a barbecue until thoroughly cooked or place the chicken in a shallow baking pan or on a cookie sheet and bake for 1 hour in an oven that has been preheated to 350°F.

To add extra crispness to oven-baked chicken, for the final 10 minutes of cooking, turn the oven temperature to broil. To avoid burning the chicken, watch it carefully.

Serve warm or cold.

VARIATIONS

Steaks and burgers take on great flavors from this marinade. Prepare the steak as you would chicken. For great Cajun barbecued burgers, add a small portion of the marinade to ground beef, form the beef into patties, and grill or broil them as usual.

Succulent Barbecued Pork Chops

PREP TIME: 15 minutes
COOK TIME: 1 hour

SERVINGS: 4
CARBS PER SERVING: 2 grams

If you love a powerful barbecue flavor, you'll enjoy these chops right off the grill. Or pop them in your broiler. Plain old oven cooking can't diminish their flavor.

1/2 stick unsalted butter
2 tablespoons soy sauce
1 teaspoon cayenne
1 teaspoon ground black pepper
1 teaspoon crushed red pepper
1 teaspoon garlic powder

2 teaspoons dried rosemary
2 teaspoons dried basil
1/2 teaspoon dried oregano
1 teaspoon salt
1/2 cup olive oil
4 pork center loin chops (about 4 to 6 ounces each)

In a large skillet, melt the butter over very low heat. Remove the skillet from the heat and allow it to cool. Add the soy sauce, mixing constantly.

Add all the spices and salt. Mix well. Return the skillet to very low heat and add the olive oil, stirring to keep the mixture from separating.

Allow the mixture to cool for 5 to 10 minutes.

Prepare the grill or preheat the oven to 350°F.

While it is still liquid, reserve half of the butter mixture for later basting. Place the chops in a skillet with the remainder of the mixture and coat the chops.

Remove the chops from the skillet and cook thoroughly on the grill or in the oven. Discard the butter mixture from the skillet.

Using only the butter mixture that did *not* make contact with uncooked pork, turn the chops and baste halfway through cooking. If you're cooking the chops in the oven, broil them during the last 10 minutes of cooking to make them crispy and brown.

Serve warm.

Campfire Chowder

PREP TIME: 25 minutes

COOK TIME: 25 minutes

SERVINGS: 4

CARBS PER SERVING: 4 grams

The smoky taste of this rich soup will satisfy your need for barbecue without your ever having to fire up the grill. We created this recipe on a fishing trip with two friends who failed to mention they hadn't brought enough backup food supplies. At the last minute, we had packed along canned clams, the only portable source of protein we had in the house. Good thing, too! When our friends failed to catch even one fish, we fried up the leftover bacon from breakfast and made a soup that was far better than any imaginary fish dinner.

1/2 pound bacon, cooked crisp and crumbled

2 tablespoons olive oil

1/4 cup diced onion

1/2 cup diced celery

1/4 pound kohlrabi, cut into 3/4-inch cubes (optional)

2 cans (6.5 ounces each) fully cooked clams, drained (retain juice) and chopped

2 cups clam juice and/or chicken stock (or our Classic Chicken Stock, page 66)

1/2 teaspoon ground black pepper

1/2 teaspoon dried thyme

1 teaspoon dried basil

1/4 teaspoon paprika, sweet or hot

Dash of cayenne (optional)

Dash of salt

1 cup heavy whipping cream

2 teaspoons arrowroot powder dissolved in 4 teaspoons of water (for thickening) (optional)

1/4 cup snipped chives, as garnish (optional)

In a skillet, fry the bacon in the olive oil until completely cooked and set it aside, discarding the bacon grease. In the same skillet, sauté the onion until translucent. Add the celery and continue to sauté until the onion browns and the celery softens.

Remove the skillet from the heat, and add the kohlrabi, clam juice and/or chicken broth, pepper, thyme, basil, paprika, cayenne, and salt. Cover and cook over low heat, stirring often, for about 10 minutes.

Turn off the heat and allow the skillet to sit for 5 minutes. Stir in

(continued)

the heavy cream and the clams. Add the bacon, crumbled, and mix. Heat slowly.

Remove from the heat. If desired, add the arrowroot and water mixture for thickening. Stir constantly to make certain it is distributed throughout.

Serve warm topped with snipped chives as garnish.

Sydney Harbor Prawns

PREP TIME: 6 minutes

COOK TIME: 10 minutes

SERVINGS: 4

CARBS PER SERVING: 2 grams

Australian barbecues are legendary to the point that Aussies write songs about them. We came across the original version of this recipe at a friend's cookout that lasted from one sunset until the next. This dish was the first course, served with great company and a red-streaked end-of-day view of Sydney's harbor. The olive oil marinade keeps the shrimp juicy. The flavor is Aussie to the core.

1/2 medium diced tomato
1 cup olive oil
1/2 cup lemon juice
1 teaspoon soy sauce
1 teaspoon salt
1 teaspoon paprika
4 teaspoons diced onion

1/2 teaspoon dried thyme
1/2 teaspoon garlic powder
1 1/2 pounds large shrimp (or prawns), cleaned, shelled, and deveined
6 romaine lettuce leaves (or arugula)

In a large, shallow bowl, combine the tomato, olive oil, lemon juice, soy sauce, salt, paprika, onion, thyme, and garlic powder. Mix well. Add the shrimp so that the marinade completely covers it.

Cover the bowl and refrigerate for 2 hours, then discard the marinade.

Fire up the barbecue grill to the appropriate temperature, or preheat the broiler.

Place the shrimp in a grill holder or on metal skewers and cook over the hot grill for 5 minutes; turn and cook an additional 5 minutes. Or broil the shrimp in the oven for 5 minutes, then turn and broil an additional 2 minutes. In either case, cook until the shrimp are opaque and thoroughly cooked.

Serve warm on a bed of lettuce or arugula.

Bacon-Wrapped Scallops

PREP TIME: 15 minutes   SERVINGS: 4
COOK TIME: 25 minutes   CARBS PER SERVING: 2 grams

We love these appetizers as a prelude to any low-carb meal. They're also great with celery stuffed with cream cheese as a change-of-pace snack.

10 strips bacon
1/4 cup soy sauce
1/4 cup water
20 medium sea scallops
20 wooden toothpicks

Olive oil or nonstick
cooking spray
Dash of cayenne or paprika
(hot or sweet) (optional)

Preheat the oven to 400°F.

Cut the bacon strips in half, crosswise. Cook the strips in a skillet until almost cooked through but not yet browned or crispy. Drain them on a paper towel, allowing them to cool completely.

Meanwhile, combine the soy sauce and water in a small bowl.

Dip each scallop into the mixture and place it on a plate. Wrap 1 half slice of cooled bacon around each scallop and secure with a toothpick.

Oil a baking pan or cookie sheet or spray one with nonstick cooking spray, then evenly space the scallops on it.

Sprinkle the scallops with a dash of cayenne or paprika and bake them in the oven until the bacon becomes crisp and the scallops are thoroughly cooked and no longer translucent (about 10 minutes).

Drain them on paper towels and serve warm or cool. Remember to remove the toothpicks before eating.

Tangy Barbecued Burgers

PREP TIME: 10 minutes
COOK TIME: 20 minutes

SERVINGS: 4
CARBS PER SERVING: 3 grams

The secret to the tang of these burgers is the combination of citrus juice and mustard. The blend of flavors complements the smoky flavor that the barbecue adds and makes the burger taste so good you'll want to make extra to enjoy cold or reheated the next day.

1 pound ground beef
1 clove garlic, minced
1 tablespoon fresh lemon juice
1 teaspoon prepared mustard
1 egg, beaten
Dash of curry powder (optional)
1 tablespoon dried basil
1 tablespoon parsley flakes
Salt and pepper, as desired

Fire up the grill or preheat the broiler. Place the beef in a large bowl. In a second smaller bowl, combine all remaining ingredients.

Using a utensil or your hands, work all the ingredients into the ground beef, making certain they are distributed evenly and well mixed.

Form the meat into four patties of equal size and grill or broil them until they are thoroughly cooked. If you prefer, cook the patties on both sides in 3 tablespoons of olive oil in a hot skillet, until they are cooked through to the center.

Serve warm topped with a slice of your favorite cheese, or cold.

VARIATIONS

Use ground turkey instead of ground beef, or in combination with ground beef or ground pork.

Perfect Low-Carb Potato Salad

PREP TIME: 15 minutes
COOK TIME: 5 minutes

SERVINGS: 4
CARBS PER SERVING: 5 grams

One summer evening we were aching for the "real thing" and decided to come up with a dish that would serve as the "next best thing." We discovered we liked the crunchy texture and caramelized onion flavor of this dish even better than the high-carb alternative. This one will surprise you!

½ head cauliflower, cut into 1-inch pieces
¼ cup diced onion
1 tablespoon olive oil
1 stalk celery, diced
2 hard-boiled eggs, chopped fine

1 cup mayonnaise (or our Instant Onion Dip, page 225)
4 strips bacon, cooked crisp and crumbled
½ teaspoon lemon pepper
½ tablespoon parsley flakes

Place the cauliflower in 2 inches of water in a medium-size pot. Cover and cook over medium heat for about 5 minutes. Do not overcook; cauliflower should be tender (a fork slips through easily) but not mushy.

While the cauliflower cooks, sauté the diced onion in olive oil in a small skillet over a medium-high flame. Continue to cook until the onion bits turn golden brown (about 3 minutes). Remove the pan from the heat. Drain the onion and discard the oil. Set the onion aside.

As soon as the cauliflower is cooked, plunge it into cold water to cool it and stop all cooking. Drain and set aside.

Place the onion, celery, chopped egg, mayonnaise, crumbled bacon, lemon pepper, and parsley flakes in a large bowl. Add the cauliflower and toss well, coating the cauliflower completely.

Cover and place in the refrigerator until thoroughly chilled.

Big Jim's Blood-in-Your-Eye Barbecue Sauce

PREP TIME: 5 minutes
COOK TIME: 5 minutes

SERVINGS: 6 (¼ cup each)
CARBS PER SERVING: 3 grams

Eastern North Carolina barbecue sauces don't depend on a tomato base, so they're perfect for low-carb dieters. Big Jim is one of the best cooks in the region. He stands five feet tall—exactly—but he makes a barbecue sauce with a powerful wallop. When folks first told us the name of his renowned sauce, we thought they mistakenly meant "mud in your eye." One taste and we knew where this marinade got its name. We've toned down the heat in our version, but we've kept all the flavor.

½ cup olive oil
¼ cup lemon juice
½ cup white vinegar
¼ cup soy sauce
1 teaspoon hot sauce

¼ teaspoon crushed red pepper
4 sardines in oil, mashed
Salt and pepper, as desired

Combine all the ingredients in a small bowl. Transfer the mixture to a small saucepan and warm it over a low flame while stirring continuously for 5 minutes. Do *not* bring to a boil.

Transfer the mixture to a small screw-top jar. Screw on the lid and store the sauce in the refrigerator. It tastes best if the flavors are left to meld for 48 hours before using. Fiery flavors increase as the sauce ages; it may be stored refrigerated for up to a week.

Shake it well immediately before using.

Classic Coleslaw

PREP TIME: 10 minutes   SERVINGS: 4
COOK TIME: 8 minutes   CARBS PER SERVING: 5 grams

Add this low-carb variety of a traditional favorite to one of our barbecue main dishes and you have an instant and legal cookout. The poppy or caraway seeds add a flavor that makes you think you're eating a sweeter, high-carb version.

2 cups shredded cabbage	2 tablespoons white vinegar
2 tablespoons chopped onion	1/2 cup mayonnaise
2 tablespoons chopped fresh parsley	2 tablespoons poppy or caraway seeds (optional)
2 slices bacon, cooked crisp and crumbled	Salt and pepper, as desired

Toss the cabbage, onion, and parsley together in a medium-size bowl. Add the bacon and vinegar and mix well. Add the mayonnaise, poppy or caraway seeds, and salt and pepper, and again mix well.

The slaw is best when covered and left in the refrigerator to chill for at least 5 hours.

Serve cold.

Grab-and-Go BBQ

PREP TIME: 10 minutes
COOK TIME: none

SERVINGS: 4
CARBS PER SERVING: 3 grams

Sometimes you crave something with a deep, smoky taste but don't have the time (or desire) to start grilling a meal. This snack takes only a few minutes to make and can be prepared a day in advance so it's ready when you are.

3 ounces cream cheese
1/2 cup sour cream
1/2 cup smoked cheddar cheese, grated
2 tablespoons Dijon mustard
6 slices bacon, cooked crisp and crumbled
1/4 cup white vinegar

1/4 cup chopped cilantro
1 tablespoon rosemary
1 tablespoon garlic powder
1/4 teaspoon ground black pepper
6 large stalks celery, cleaned but whole

With a mixer or blender, process together the cream cheese, sour cream, cheese, and mustard until smooth. Add the bacon, vinegar, herbs and seasonings and blend thoroughly.

Stuff the mixture into the celery stalks, cover each stalk with plastic wrap, and chill well.

Maggie's Magic Eggs

PREP TIME: 10 minutes
COOK TIME: 2 to 3 minutes

SERVINGS: 4
CARBS PER SERVING: 2 grams

In a small hostel in Rotorua, New Zealand, about three blocks from the central bus station lives Margaret Pollet, one of our favorite self-taught chefs. Maggie claims to be ninety-two (and we wouldn't think of challenging the point), and to this day, she does all the cooking every day for a dozen hungry travelers. When our planned barbecue had to be cancelled because of rain, Maggie came to the rescue with a barbecue-flavored treat that disappeared even as she tried to get the platter to the table. Here's our own low-carb version.

2 teaspoons chopped onion
1 tablespoon olive oil (more, if needed)
4 hard-boiled eggs, peeled
1/8 teaspoon ground rosemary
1/8 teaspoon ground basil
Dash of salt
Dash of ground black pepper
2 sausage patties, fully cooked, crumbled (or our Freedom Sausage, page 23, fully cooked, crumbled)
Dash of hot sauce

In a small saucepan over medium heat, sauté the onion in the olive oil, stirring constantly until it browns (2 to 3 minutes). Remove the pan from the heat and set it aside.

Split the hard-boiled eggs in half and remove the yolks to a small bowl.

Add the rosemary, basil, and salt, pepper and crumbled sausage to the yolks and mix well.

Add the sautéed onion bits and thin the mixture with pan drippings (or additional olive oil as needed) until it becomes a thick paste.

Fill the egg white halves with the mixture.

Serve immediately with hot sauce, or chill first.

Freedom Sausage

PREP TIME: 10 minutes
COOK TIME: 20 minutes

SERVINGS: 4 (12 patties)
CARBS PER SERVING: 1 gram

We have become friends with many of the cast members at the Tokyo Disney Resort and were honored to be invited to their private cast party. The get-together happened to take place on July 4, and to make us feel at home they served sausage barbecued on a hibachi. The powerful Eastern flavor kept us coming back for more. Although we've replaced the rice in the original dish with low-carb pork rinds, we bet you'll love our version of this dish, too.

1 pound ground pork
1/2 pound ground beef
2 teaspoons lemon juice
1 teaspoon fresh ginger root, peeled and finely grated (optional)

1 teaspoon prepared wasabi (or white prepared horseradish, or hot sauce)
1/2 teaspoon salt
2 eggs
1 cup crushed pork rinds

Fire up the grill.

Combine all the ingredients in a large mixing bowl. Mix well.

Form the mixture into 12 patties and grill them until thoroughly cooked. Alternatively, the patties may be fried in 2 tablespoons of olive oil in a large skillet over a medium flame. Fry each patty for about 6 minutes in hot (but not smoking) oil, until brown and cooked throughout.

VARIATIONS

Smoky Flavored Sausage: add a few drops of liquid smoke flavoring (available in the barbecue section of the supermarket).

Old-Fashioned Sausage: substitute 1 teaspoon dried sage for the ginger root.

Kebabs with a Kick

PREP TIME: 10 minutes

COOK TIME: 12 minutes

SERVINGS: 4

CARBS PER SERVING: 5 grams

The kick in this great barbecue comes from the lemon juice, soy sauce, and crushed red pepper exploding with flavor when they are heated. Allowing the meat to marinate in the refrigerator allows the good flavor to saturate every mouthful.

Juice from 1/2 lemon (seeds removed)
2 tablespoons olive oil
1 teaspoon soy sauce
3 cloves garlic, finely chopped
1/2 teaspoon crushed red pepper

1 pound lamb, cut into kebab-size cubes (11/2 inches)
2 green bell peppers, cut into 11/2-inch-square pieces
8 mushroom caps

Combine the lemon juice, olive oil, soy sauce, garlic, and crushed red pepper in a large pot. Stir the mixture and cook very slowly over a low flame until it becomes warm, not hot.

Remove the pot from the heat.

Add the lamb, green peppers, and mushroom caps. Coat them well. Cover the mixture and chill it in the refrigerator for two hours, stirring several times.

Remove the meat and vegetables and discard the marinade.

Thread the meat cubes onto metal skewers, alternating them with slices of green pepper and mushrooms.

Grill the kebabs for about 8 minutes on each side until the meat and vegetables are thoroughly cooked. Turn the kebabs frequently to ensure even cooking.

CHEESE-FILLED TREATS

Almost No-Carb Parmesan Puffs

PREP TIME: 3 minutes
COOK TIME: 8 minutes

SERVINGS: 2 (3 puffs each)
CARBS PER SERVING: ¼ gram

We can't wait to share these gems! They're fast, easy, and require only three ingredients that most people have handy. Plus, they're delicious, and contain almost no carbs!

2 egg whites
¼ cup grated Parmesan cheese

½ cup olive oil

Place the egg whites in a dry mixing bowl and beat them with an electric mixer at medium speed until stiff peaks are formed.

Gently fold in the Parmesan cheese, using a tablespoon so that the egg white peaks are disturbed as little as possible.

In a large skillet over a medium flame, heat the olive oil until hot (but not smoking).

Drop 6 equal dollops of the egg white mixture into the hot oil. Do not disturb the puffs until the edges begin to brown.

When the puffs are well browned on one side (about 5 minutes), turn them gently, using a spatula and a spoon, and cook them until they're golden brown on the other side (another 3 minutes). Make certain that all surfaces are well browned.

Remove each puff to a plate and serve it warm or cold.

Serve these puffs with our Four-Spice Creamy Dip (page 273) or one of our homemade hot sauces (pages 259–261), or enjoy them all by themselves.

VARIATIONS

Add a dash of cayenne pepper along with the Parmesan cheese for a spicy, cheesy pop-em.

Or fold finely grated American cheese into the stiffened egg whites in place of grated Parmesan. The puffs will be a bit less puffy but the savory-cheesy taste is terrific.

For a thicker, chewier puff, in addition to the cheese, add ¼ cup pork rinds that have been crumbled to the texture of bread crumbs.

No Worries Caesar Salad

PREP TIME: 10 minutes	SERVINGS: 4
COOK TIME: none	CARBS PER SERVING: 3 grams

While traveling on Kangaroo Island in Australia (where there are more koalas than kangaroos), we were concerned about the safety of eating raw (or lightly cooked) eggs, so we refrained from enjoying our beloved Caesar salads. Once we returned home, that experience inspired us to seek a substitute for the raw egg traditionally added to a Caesar. The mixture we discovered actually makes for a smoother, creamier base for the fragrant Parmesan cheese in this classic delight.

1 teaspoon kosher salt for sprinkling (optional)
2 cloves garlic, peeled and sliced in half
1/2 teaspoon dry mustard
2 teaspoons lemon juice
Dash of hot sauce
4 tablespoons olive oil

6 cups torn and chilled lettuce leaves (romaine, Bibb, leaf, or arugula)
4 tablespoons grated Parmesan cheese
6 anchovies in oil, drained and mashed
2 tablespoons mayonnaise

Sprinkle the salt in the bottom of a large wooden salad bowl. Rub the garlic cloves around the inside of the bowl, tearing them against the salt.

Add the mustard, lemon juice, and hot sauce. Stir the mixture to combine and dissolve the salt. Whisk in 2 tablespoons of the olive oil (reserve the other 2 tablespoons of oil). Stir briskly to blend the ingredients. Add the torn lettuce leaves to the bowl and toss them to coat with the salt, garlic, and oil mixture. Sprinkle the salad mix with the Parmesan cheese and add the anchovies.

In a small jar, combine the mayonnaise with the remaining 2 tablespoons of olive oil. Cover the jar and shake the mixture very well. Pour the mayonnaise-oil dressing quickly over the salad, tossing gently but thoroughly to bring up all the good cheese and anchovies on the bottom of the bowl.

Winter Night Tuna Melt

PREP TIME: 12 minutes

COOK TIME: 5 minutes

SERVINGS: 4

CARBS PER SERVING: 5 grams

Rachael: *Before I met Richard, I lost 165 pounds in two years using the program we outline in our books* The Carbohydrate Addict's LifeSpan Program *and* The Carbohydrate Addict's 7-Day Plan. *Cold winter nights were the hard times. I longed for something warm and comfy and, of course, high in carbs. Here's the solution that helped me make it through. Now Richard and I enjoy this dish together, no matter what the time of year.*

4 large tomatoes
2 tablespoons olive oil
1/2 cup sour cream
1/4 cup chopped cucumber
1/4 cup diced green bell pepper
1/4 cup diced scallions
1 teaspoon dried basil
1/4 teaspoon garlic powder

1 can (6 1/2 ounces) tuna, packed in water, drained and flaked
4 to 8 thick slices (3 to 6 ounces) cheese (cheddar, American, Swiss, or Monterey Jack), grated
6 leaves lettuce (Bibb, romaine, leaf, or arugula)

Place the tomatoes on a well-oiled baking sheet.

In a medium-size bowl, combine the sour cream, cucumber, green pepper, scallions, basil, and garlic powder. Mix well. Stir in the tuna and mix again. Set the mixture aside.

Scoop out the insides of each tomato, discarding the seeds and liquid, leaving only shells.

Spoon the tuna mixture into the center of each tomato shell.

Top each shell with one or two slices of cheese and bake at 350°F for three to five minutes (or until the cheese is fully melted). If desired, place the tomatoes under the broiler for a minute or two to crisp the cheese, but watch carefully to prevent burning.

Serve warm on several large lettuce or arugula leaves.

VARIATIONS

Sprinkle the tuna melt with Parmesan or Romano cheese, as desired, right before adding cheese slices on top.

(*continued*)

Stuff the tuna mixture into green pepper shells instead of tomato shells (this reduces the carb count by 2 grams).

Use cooked, diced chicken, turkey, beef, or pork instead of tuna.

Quick Carbonara

PREP TIME: 10 minutes
COOK TIME: 20 minutes

SERVINGS: 4
CARBS PER SERVING: 4 grams

Sometimes you want something that tastes like barbecue but you don't feel like an all-meat dish. This recipe will give you the taste without the grill.

8 slices bacon
1/2 small onion, chopped
1 clove garlic, minced
1 pound fresh green beans (or snap beans), cleaned OR
1 1/2 bags (10 ounces each) frozen green beans
4 eggs
3 tablespoons heavy whipping cream

1/2 teaspoon crushed red pepper (or dash of hot sauce)
1 teaspoon paprika, hot or sweet
Salt and pepper, as desired
1/2 cup grated Romano or Parmesan cheese
4 slices (3 to 4 ounces) smoky cheddar or jalapeño cheese

In a medium-size nonstick skillet over a medium flame, fry the bacon until the meat begins to brown and the grease has been released. Add the onion and garlic and continue to cook until the bacon is fully cooked (but not crisp) and the onion turns translucent. Stir often to prevent sticking. Remove the skillet from the heat to cool.

Place the green beans in 2 tablespoons of water in a 2-quart microwave-safe container.

Cover the container and microwave on high for 10 minutes, stirring twice during cooking.

While the beans are cooking, drain all but about 1 tablespoon of the bacon fat from the skillet. Remove the bacon, dice it, and return it to the skillet with the onion mixture. Return the skillet to low heat and warm slightly.

While the bacon warms, beat together the eggs, cream, crushed red pepper (or hot sauce), paprika, and salt and pepper as desired.

Raise the heat under the skillet to medium and add the egg mixture, hot green beans, and Parmesan or Romano cheese, stirring until the eggs are thoroughly cooked.

Top with the cheese slices, turn off the heat, cover, and allow the carbonara to stand for two minutes or until the cheese slices melt.

Serve immediately.

Chewy Cheesy Mozzarella Logs

PREP TIME: 10 minutes
COOK TIME: 10 minutes

SERVINGS: 4
CARBS PER SERVING: 1 gram

When the day's work is done, when everyone else's needs have been taken care of, we know we can always relax with this great late-night snack.

2 cups crushed pork rinds
1/4 teaspoon ground black pepper
1/2 teaspoon dried oregano
1 teaspoon paprika, hot or sweet

1 egg
1/4 cup olive oil
8 sticks (1 ounce each) mozzarella cheese

In a blender, food processor, or by hand, crumble and combine the pork rinds, pepper, oregano, and paprika. Remove the mixture to a shallow dish.

In another shallow dish, beat the egg until it's foamy.

Heat the oil in a medium-size frying pan over medium heat until the oil is hot (but not smoking).

Dip the coated cheese sticks first into the egg, then into the pork rind mixture. Fry the sticks over medium heat, turning often, until they are golden brown.

Serve warm.

Silky-Smooth Cheese Sauce

PREP TIME: 10 minutes

COOK TIME: 6 minutes

SERVINGS: 4

CARBS PER SERVING: 1 gram

We always cook more meat or chicken than we'll need at a meal. Leftovers add variety to the next meal and give a ready answer to the eternal question "What can I have as a low-carb snack?" This sauce is a favorite. It turns any leftover into an instant meal or treat.

4   mushroom caps, sliced
1/4   cup diced scallions
2   tablespoons unsalted butter
1/4   cup heavy whipping cream
1/2   teaspoon fresh basil

1/2   teaspoon ground black pepper
1/4   teaspoon cayenne
1   cup grated cheese (cheddar, American, Swiss, or Monterey Jack)

Sauté the mushroom caps and scallions in butter in a medium-size skillet over medium heat until soft, about 4 minutes. Drain them well and remove them to a small bowl.

Make the sauce by heating the cream in a saucepan over a medium flame. Heat it until bubbles begin to form around the outside, but do not allow the cream to boil.

Add the basil, pepper, and cayenne. Stir.

Reduce to a very low heat and mix in the cheese a bit at a time, stirring continuously. Add mushroom-scallion mixture.

Immediately pour the sauce over leftover meat, chicken, or steamed vegetables.

Do not attempt to reheat or store this sauce, as it will break down and become inedible.

Savory Tarts

PREP TIME: 10 minutes
COOK TIME: 30 to 35 minutes

SERVINGS: 16 tarts
CARBS PER SERVING: 1 gram

In Australia and New Zealand, morning muffins are often more savory than sweet. We love the flavor in this low-carb version.

8 ounces ground beef
2 tablespoons chopped onion
1 teaspoon pressed garlic
1 tablespoon olive oil
3 egg whites
1 egg
1/2 cup crushed pork rinds

1 tablespoon minced fresh parsley
1/4 teaspoon dried dill
1/8 teaspoon cayenne
1 cup grated mozzarella cheese
1/4 cup ricotta cheese

Preheat the oven to 350°F. Lightly oil a baking sheet.

In a heavy skillet over medium-high heat, sauté the ground beef, onion, and garlic in the olive oil until the meat is slightly browned. Put the skillet aside.

In a medium-size mixing bowl, beat the egg whites until soft peaks are formed. Set them aside.

In a separate medium-size mixing bowl, beat the whole egg. Add the crushed pork rinds, parsley, dill, cayenne, and cheeses. Add the sautéed beef mixture. Mix well.

Gently fold the beef mixture into the beaten egg whites, a bit at a time, so that the peaks are not eliminated.

Turn this mixture onto the oiled baking sheet and spread evenly into a rectangle.

Bake until the mixture has set (25 to 30 minutes). Let it cool, then cut it into squares.

Serve warm or cold.

Midnight Pizza

PREP TIME: 15 minutes
COOK TIME: 20 to 25 minutes

SERVINGS: 9-inch pizza (serves 2)
CARBS PER SERVING: 4 grams

This recipe has a terrifically low carb count yet fully satisfies. The perfect solution for nights when you absolutely must have a yummy snack.

Pizza Base

4 eggs
3 ounces cream cheese, cut into 1-inch blocks, softened

2 tablespoons grated Romano or Parmesan cheese
Nonstick cooking spray

Pizza Topping

12 ripe black olives, drained, pitted, and sliced
1/2 tomato, diced and drained of all liquid

4 ounces shredded mozzarella cheese
1 clove garlic, pressed (or 1/2 teaspoon garlic powder)
1/2 teaspoon oregano

Preheat the oven to 350°F.

Pizza base: In a medium-size bowl, combine the eggs, cream cheese, and Romano or Parmesan cheese. Mix well. (Some cream cheese lumps may remain).

Spray a 9-inch pie pan with nonstick cooking spray and pour in the base mixture.

Bake for 10 to 15 minutes or until the base begins to set. Allow it to cool until firmly set.

Pizza topping: Cover the cooled base with a layer of sliced olives, followed by a layer each of diced tomato and shredded mozzarella. Season with garlic and oregano.

Bake the pizza for another 10 minutes at 350°F. Allow it to remain cooling in the pie pan for an additional 5 to 10 minutes before serving warm.

VARIATION

Before adding mozzarella to the pizza topping, add leftover cooked

(continued)

and diced beef, pork, or chicken and/or precooked low-carb vegetables. Add mozzarella, garlic, and oregano and bake for 15 minutes at 350°F, then cool and serve as above.

Velvety Cheese Soufflé

PREP TIME: 12 minutes

COOK TIME: 1 hour

SERVINGS: 9-inch soufflé (serves 4)

CARBS PER SERVING: 1 gram

Rachael: *Every six months or so, my friend, Gayle, and I used to meet at a restaurant and share a low-carb breakfast and a couple of hours of nonstop catching up. The only problem was Gayle's inability to get anyplace on time. I'd wait at the restaurant for a half hour, sometimes an hour, before she'd come rushing through the door with a heap of apologies and excuses. I solved the problem by inviting her to my home for breakfast and serving up this wonderful soufflé that is ready no matter when she arrives.*

Olive oil to grease the inside of a 9-inch pie pan

1 cup light whipping cream

1 cup grated cheese (cheddar or American)

1½ teaspoons dried basil

½ teaspoon paprika (hot or sweet)

4 eggs

Salt and pepper, as desired

Preheat the oven to 325°F.

Oil the sides and bottom of a 9-inch pie pan.

In a medium-size saucepan, heat the cream until it is scalded. Watch carefully so it does not boil over. Reduce heat and stir in the grated cheese. When the cheese is melted, add the basil and paprika.

Remove the pan from the heat. Allow the mixture to cool for 6 minutes. Add 1 egg at a time, mixing thoroughly until all the eggs are incorporated. Season with salt and pepper, as desired, and mix well.

Pour the mixture into the pie pan, place the pan in the oven, and bake until the soufflé center is set and solid (40 to 50 minutes).

Serve warm or cold.

Canadian Cheese Soup

PREP TIME: 35 minutes
COOK TIME: 30 minutes

SERVINGS: 2
CARBS PER SERVING: 4 grams

At EPCOT in Disney World, the Canadian pavilion serves up a cheese soup that makes us groan with pleasure. We put together this low-carb adaptation of their superb soup and it works beautifully! It's very rich, so we save it for special occasions.

1/4 pound bacon, cut into
   1/2-inch pieces
2 tablespoons unsalted butter
1 stalk celery, diced
1/2 small red onion, diced
2 cups light whipping cream
1 cup grated cheddar cheese
   Dash of hot sauce

Salt and pepper
2 teaspoons arrowroot
   powder dissolved in
   4 teaspoons of water, for
   thickening (optional)
2 tablespoons chopped
   scallions, parsley, or chives
   (optional)

In a soup pot, brown the bacon over medium heat. As the bacon begins to crisp, transfer it to a paper towel to drain. Melt the butter and sauté the celery and onion in the pot until the onion softens, stirring often. Add the cream and simmer for 15 minutes. Do not allow the mixture to boil.

Turn off heat and stir in the cheese, followed by the hot sauce, and salt and pepper as desired. Stir well, until all the cheese is melted.

If desired, add the arrowroot and water mixture for thickening. Stir constantly to make certain it is distributed throughout.

Top with chopped scallions, parsley, or chives and serve warm.

Green Pepper with Cheese Dip

PREP TIME: 35 minutes

COOK TIME: 10 minutes

SERVINGS: 2

CARBS PER SERVING: 1 gram

After visiting the Arc de Triomphe, the Eiffel Tower, and the Champs Élysées in the same morning, we were more than ready for lunch at one of the renowned Parisian restaurants. Sadly, we discovered that all the fine restaurants were closed up tight until evening. A little café on Rue de MacMahon came to the rescue, offering an array of exciting delicacies we could munch on while watching the world go by and resting our weary feet. Here's our low-carb version of their much-appreciated dip (which used duck instead of bacon). Serve this one with a variety of low-carb vegetables for perfect crudités.

1 large green bell pepper
2 strips bacon
1 cup grated cheddar cheese, extra sharp
1/2 cup mayonnaise
1 tablespoon diced onion
1 tablespoon white prepared horseradish

3 cups raw low-carb vegetables (for dipping), including green beans, wax beans, snap beans, celery sticks, green pepper wedges, mushroom caps, cauliflower florets, and cucumber slices

Cut one end off the green pepper to make a wide opening, then seed and core the green pepper, leaving the shell intact to hold the dip you are about to make. Set the shell aside, uncovered, in the refrigerator.

In a small skillet on medium-high heat, fry the bacon until it is crisp. Drain it on a paper towel.

Dice the bacon and transfer it to a medium-size bowl. Add 1 tablespoon of bacon drippings from the skillet and stir well to coat the bacon. Add the cheese, mayonnaise, onion, and horseradish. Mix well.

Refrigerate the dip, covered, for 2 hours.

Meanwhile, on a large, round plate, clean, cut, and assemble a circle of raw, low-carb vegetables.

Spoon the dip into the cold green pepper shell, place it in the center of the ring of raw veggies, and serve.

Chicken Provençal

PREP TIME: 20 minutes
COOK TIME: 50 minutes

SERVINGS: 4
CARBS PER SERVING: 2 grams

A rainy day with no clearing in sight left us feeling bored and restless. When dinnertime finally came, we gathered up almost everything we had in the refrigerator and came up with this rich, gourmet-style meal that has since become a favorite. As we sat enjoying our invention, we suddenly realized we had reinvented the standard combination of herbs and ingredients that defines the signature French Provençal dish.

4 tablespoons olive oil
1 teaspoon sesame oil
4 small chicken breast halves (boneless and skinless), pounded thin for rolling
1 teaspoon soy sauce
1 clove garlic, minced
1/2 cup minced scallions
1 cup mushroom caps, cleaned and sliced

2 tablespoons chopped fresh parsley
1 teaspoon dried basil
   Black pepper, as desired
1 chunk (4 ounces) mozzarella cheese, quartered lengthwise
   Wooden toothpicks

Preheat the oven to 350°F.

Brush a cookie sheet with 1 tablespoon of the olive oil.

In a large skillet, heat the sesame oil and the remaining 3 tablespoons olive oil. Brown the chicken on one side, then flip it and brown it on the other side. Remove the pan from the heat and transfer the chicken to a cool plate.

In the same skillet, to the remaining oil add the soy sauce and heat it over a low-medium flame. Add the garlic and scallions. Cook for 3 minutes, until the scallions are soft.

Add the mushrooms and cook, stirring to prevent sticking, until they are soft, about 4 minutes.

Remove the pan from the heat. Add the parsley, basil, and black pepper as desired.

Place one quarter of the mushroom mixture and 1 piece of the mozzarella on the narrow end of one chicken breast and roll the

(continued)

chicken with the mushroom mixture and cheese inside. Secure it with wooden toothpicks, then repeat the process with the other 3 chicken breast halves.

Place the rolls onto the oiled cookie sheet, seam side down, and bake for 40 minutes, or until cooked throughout.

Remove the toothpicks and serve warm.

Four-Cheese Veggie Stuffer

PREP TIME: 8 minutes
COOK TIME: none

SERVINGS: 8 (½ cup each)
CARBS PER SERVING: 2 grams

Everyone is always asking us for quick low-carb recipes they can enjoy on the run. We've given up trying to convince them that meals were meant to be enjoyed and that they have a right to that pleasure. Bending to pressure, we've discovered a middle ground: a quick-fix, on-the-go recipe that's rich and satisfying.

3   ounces cream cheese, cut into 1-inch cubes, softened
¼   cup unsalted butter, room temperature
4   tablespoons sour cream
2   ounces feta cheese, crumbled
2   ounces grated cheese (cheddar, American, Swiss, or Monterey Jack)

2   ounces grated smoky cheddar or jalapeño cheese
1   tablespoon prepared mustard
2   tablespoons dried basil
1   teaspoon spicy (hot) paprika (optional)
½   teaspoon capers
    Vegetable for stuffing or dipping

Mix together the cream cheese and butter. Add the sour cream, feta and other cheeses, mustard, basil, and paprika. Mix well.

Stuff the mixture into celery sticks or mushroom caps or use it as a dip for raw green beans, wax beans, snap beans, cauliflower, or green pepper wedges.

Sprinkle with capers.

Best served ice cold.

Mushroom-Brie Omelet

PREP TIME: 10 minutes

COOK TIME: 12 minutes

SERVINGS: 2

CARBS PER SERVING: 3 grams

Richard: *We had been on a publicity tour for more than a month, visiting a new city and meeting readers almost every day. We arrived home happy but tired and, most of all, hungry. Making a complicated dinner was the last thing on our minds, so as I unpacked our bags, Rachael threw this dish together. "It smells like home and feels like home. I just wanted it to taste like home," she explained. And it did.*

4 ounces Brie cheese
2 tablespoons unsalted butter
4 eggs, lightly beaten
2 scallions, thinly sliced
1 jar (6 ounces) sliced
   mushrooms, drained

1/2 teaspoon crushed red
   pepper or hot sauce
   (optional)
Salt and pepper, as desired

Preheat the oven to 200°F.

Place a large ovenproof serving platter in the oven and heat it.

Trim the rind from the Brie and discard it. Slice the cheese thinly.

In a medium-size nonstick skillet over medium heat, melt the butter. Rotate the skillet to coat the bottom.

Crack the eggs into a medium-size bowl and whisk them until they're foamy.

Pour the eggs into the skillet. Let them cook, without stirring, 2 to 3 minutes, or until they are set on the bottom. With a spatula, lift the side of the omelet and slightly tilt the pan to allow the uncooked portion of egg to flow to the other side. Cover the pan and cook an additional 2 to 3 minutes, until the eggs are cooked throughout.

Remove the serving platter from the oven and slide the omelet into the center of it. Evenly space the cheese slices over one half of the omelet. Sprinkle with the scallions, mushroom slices, red pepper, and salt and pepper as desired. Flip the empty side of the omelet over the cheese-covered side to make a semicircular sandwich.

Return the platter to the oven for 2 to 3 minutes. Serve warm. Excellent with crunchy raw green beans, wax beans, or snap beans.

CHINESE DELIGHTS

Gansu Pulled Pork

PREP TIME: 15 minutes

COOK TIME: 2 hours

SERVINGS: 4

CARBS PER SERVING: 5 grams

This dish requires lots of ingredients but very little work. It's so good, you may want to double the recipe.

1 pound pork butt (this will give you the stringiest meat)

4 tablespoons soy sauce

2 tablespoons water

1 teaspoon ground black pepper

1 teaspoon paprika (hot or sweet)

1/2 teaspoon dry mustard

1/4 teaspoon cayenne (optional)

1 teaspoon grated orange zest

1 tablespoon orange juice

1 tablespoon lemon juice

1 tablespoon white vinegar

2 teaspoons soy sauce

1/2 teaspoon Dijon mustard

1/4 cup peanut oil

1 teaspoon sesame oil

Preheat the oven to 375°F.

Insert a meat thermometer into the thickest part of the pork butt and set the meat on a rack in a deep roasting pan with 1 1/2 inches of water in the bottom.

Combine the soy sauce and water in a small bowl and pour the mixture over all the exposed surfaces of the pork.

In a small bowl combine the pepper, paprika, dry mustard, and cayenne as a rub. Lift the pork and rub the mixture onto all its surfaces. Return the pork to the roasting pan.

Place the pan in the oven and roast the pork for about 2 hours (to make the meat very stringy), turning it several times so that all the surfaces have been on the bottom. Replenish the water on the bottom of the roasting pan as necessary.

When the meat has reached an internal temperature of at least 170°F, remove the pan from the oven and allow the meat to cool.

Cut off small fist-size sections of the pork and separate them into strings of meat. Pile the strings onto a cool plate.

Whisk the orange zest, orange juice, lemon juice, vinegar, soy sauce, and mustard together in a small bowl. While whisking constantly,

(continued)

slowly drizzle in both oils. Continue whisking until all the ingredients are completely blended. Transfer the oil mixture to a large skillet and heat until it is very hot but not smoking. Add the strings of pork to the skillet and coat the meat well with the oil mixture.

Stir-fry on medium heat for 5 to 7 minutes.

Serve warm. Leftovers gain even more flavor when they are refrigerated overnight.

VARIATION

While stir-frying the meat in the skillet, add your favorite low-carb vegetables, including daikon, celery, green bell pepper, and cauliflower. Cook and stir until the vegetables are as tender as you wish.

Nearly Nine Dragons
Lemon Shrimp

PREP TIME: 10 minutes

COOK TIME: 7 minutes

SERVINGS: 4

CARBS PER SERVING: 3 grams

One of our favorite restaurants at Disney World is the Nine Dragons at the EPCOT pavilion. For many years the chef offered a wonderful shrimp dish that had the best lemon sauce we had ever tasted. When the restaurant added a full menu of dim sum, some of the classic dishes had to go and their lemon sauce shrimp was one of them. This recipe is our adaptation of the Nine Dragons' wonderful creation.

1/8 cup chopped fresh parsley
1/2 teaspoon grated lemon peel
 2 cups cauliflower florets
 2 tablespoons butter
 2 cloves minced garlic
 2 tablespoons lemon juice

1 pound shrimp, fully cooked, cleaned, shelled, and deveined
Lemon slices, as garnish (optional)

Place 1 tablespoon of the parsley, the lemon peel, and about 1 inch of water in a large saucepan. Add the cauliflower and bring to a boil over medium heat. Cover and steam for 4 minutes. The cauliflower should be cooked but firm.

Transfer the cauliflower to a large bowl and cover to keep it warm, reserving and setting aside just 1/4 cup of the hot cooking liquid.

Heat the butter in a small saucepan over medium heat. Add the garlic and sauté for 1 to 2 minutes. Stir in the lemon juice and reserved cooking liquid. Remove the pan from the heat. Add the shrimp and coat well. Return the pan to the heat for 1 minute or less to heat the shrimp.

Spoon the shrimp and lemon sauce over the cauliflower. Sprinkle with the remaining parsley and toss well. Garnish with lemon slices or more parsley if desired.

VARIATION

When the shrimp is added to the lemon sauce, also add bamboo shoots, precooked mushrooms, or daikon.

Szechuan Chicken

PREP TIME: 15 minutes
COOK TIME: 25 minutes

SERVINGS: 4
CARBS PER SERVING: 4 grams

Both Hunan and Szechuan styles of Chinese cooking are famous for their fiery dishes. Hunan cuisine is often hotter than Szechuan. Both schools believe that hot peppers dry out and cool down the body, making it easier to handle the heat and humidity of their respective regions. This recipe can be adjusted to your need for heat by adding as much (or as little) of the chili peppers as you prefer. Fiery or mild, hot or cold, this dish will satisfy your craving for Chinese.

1 pound boneless, skinless chicken breasts, cut into 1/4-inch strips

4 tablespoons olive oil, divided in half

1/2 teaspoon salt

1 leek, chopped

1 to 2 teaspoon(s) fresh red or green chili peppers*, cored and cut into 1/8-inch strips

1 tablespoon soy sauce

In a large skillet or wok, stir-fry the chicken strips in half the oil for 20 minutes or until they are thoroughly cooked. Transfer the chicken with a slotted spatula to a bowl, leaving the drippings in the pan.

When the chicken has cooled, add the salt to the chicken strips with your fingers. Stir and mix to make sure the chicken is well coated.

Add the remaining oil to the skillet or wok and heat over a medium-high flame.

Stir-fry the leek and chili peppers, quickly stirring for no more than 1 to 2 minutes, to retain crispness.

Add the soy sauce and the chicken. Toss the mixture well and stir-fry together for 2 to 3 minutes.

Serve hot. Also great as a cold leftover the next day.

* NOTE: When handling chili peppers, it's always a good idea to wear rubber or latex gloves. The pepper can burn and irritate your hands even if you are not aware of any tiny cuts or abrasions that may exist. Be certain not to touch your face or eyes or any other area that may be vulnerable to damage or irritation. Immediately wash the knife, cutting surfaces, and gloves when finished.

Tibetan Stir-Fry

PREP TIME: 10 minutes   SERVINGS: 4

COOK TIME: 3 to 4 minutes   CARBS PER SERVING: approximately 3 grams, depending on the vegetables selected

Most people don't think of Tibet when they think of Chinese food, but that's where some of the world's best Chinese-style recipes originated. A good friend of ours spends summers in Tibet, where she receives spiritual guidance. She works sixty hours a week in New York during the rest of the year to be able to afford her instruction. In keeping with her work schedule and her vegetarian lifestyle, her low-carb diet must include recipes that are quick, tasty, and non-meat. We helped her develop this one, and we liked it so much, we often make it for ourselves, either with tofu or as a side to our meat or chicken dishes.

2 tablespoons olive oil

1/2 teaspoon sesame oil

1 tablespoon peeled and finely grated fresh ginger root

1 clove garlic, minced

2 cups total of any of the following vegetables: sliced mushrooms, daikon, bamboo shoots, green beans, wax beans, snap beans, sliced celery, cauliflower florets, sliced green or purple cabbage, bamboo shoots, green bell pepper strips, or diced scallions

2 tablespoons soy sauce

1 teaspoon lemon juice

Heat the olive oil, sesame oil, and ginger in a wok or large skillet.

Add the garlic and vegetables, and quickly stir-fry until just barely tender (3 to 4 minutes). Stir in the soy sauce and lemon juice. Mix well and cover. Remove from heat. Allow the dish to sit for a few moments, so that flavors can meld before serving.

Fujian Duck

PREP TIME: 10 minutes

COOK TIME: 2 to 2½ hours

SERVINGS: 4

CARBS PER SERVING: 2 grams

This interesting combination of flavors comes from Fujian, a Chinese province that is home to more than 27 million people. Even so, we had never heard of it, but after enjoying the powerful tastes of the region, we will never forget it.

½ cup olive oil

½ teaspoon fresh red or green chili peppers, seeded and finely diced (or ¼ teaspoon crushed red pepper)

1 clove garlic, minced

1 scallion, minced

3 sprigs fresh coriander, stems only, diced finely

½ teaspoon peeled and finely grated fresh ginger root

½ teaspoon sesame oil

1 duckling (approximately 2 pounds)

Preheat the oven to 350°F.

In a medium-size saucepan over medium-low heat, heat the olive oil until it is warm but not smoking (around 300°F). Pour the oil into a bowl.

Add the chili pepper, garlic, scallion, coriander, and ginger root. Stir well. Add the sesame oil. Mix well again. Allow to cool to room temperature.

Pour the mixture into the palm of your hand, then smear it all over the duck.

Into a deep roasting pan pour 1 inch of water. Place the duck on a rack in the pan. Insert a meat thermometer into the thickest part of the duck breast, away from any bone.

Roast the duck for 2 to 2½ hours, or until the temperature gauge on the meat thermometer indicates an internal temperature of 185°F. Add water to the bottom of the roasting pan as needed during the cooking process.

Allow the duck to cool for 10 minutes before carving. Serve it warm with the au jus gravy from the bottom of the roasting pan.

This dish goes well with salad and vegetables. It's also great cold as a snack.

Simple Egg Drop Soup

PREP TIME: 5 minutes
COOK TIME: 1½ minutes

SERVINGS: 4
CARBS PER SERVING: 3 grams

As good as in a restaurant, with little work and almost no carbs.

1 quart chicken stock (Classic
  Chicken Stock, Chinese
  variation, page 67)
2 tablespoons soy sauce

½ cup sliced scallion, green
  and white parts
4 eggs, beaten lightly

Combine the chicken stock, soy sauce, and scallion in a large saucepan. Bring to a boil.

Very slowly, pour the beaten eggs in a steady stream into the boiling broth to form ribbons of egg. Cook for 1½ minutes.

Serve immediately.

Classic Chop Suey

PREP TIME: 10 minutes
COOK TIME: 20 minutes

SERVINGS: 4
CARBS PER SERVING: 3 grams

We had only an hour to make dinner, eat it, and get dressed for an event, and we were both really craving Chinese food. Fortunately, we had the makings for this invention on hand. Now we pre-cube and freeze the chicken and pork so we can whip up this recipe at a moment's notice.

½ pound chicken, cut into 1-inch cubes
½ pound pork, cut into 1-inch cubes
4 tablespoons peanut oil
2 stalks celery, diced

½ cup canned bamboo shoots, drained and thinly sliced
½ cup daikon, thinly sliced
1 teaspoon soy sauce
Salt and pepper, as desired
Stir-fried cabbage or grated daikon as a serving bed

Stir-fry the chicken and pork cubes in the peanut oil over medium heat, in a large skillet or wok. Cook, stirring constantly, until all the meat is white and thoroughly cooked (about 20 minutes).

Add the celery, bamboo shoots, daikon, soy sauce, and salt and pepper as desired. Stir-fry over medium heat for 3 minutes.

Serve over crisp sautéed cabbage or grated daikon.

Kiwi Green Pepper Steak

PREP TIME: 15 minutes

COOK TIME: 25 minutes

SERVINGS: 4

CARBS PER SERVING: 4 grams

Picture this: You're in Auckland, New Zealand, and you've had lamb for the last three days. What you really want is something Chinese, but where in the world can you get it? The answer: in Auckland's famous Chinatown! Restaurants by the dozen, each better than the last, with fine food and much of it low-carb adaptable. Many New Zealanders call themselves Kiwis, so our version of this great New Zealand (aka Chinese) dish is named in their honor.

1 pound steak, rib eye or strip without bone, cut into 1/2-inch strips
3 tablespoons olive oil
1 tablespoon sesame oil
2 cloves garlic, diced
2 tablespoons soy sauce
1/2 cup scallions, sliced
1 cup green bell pepper, cut into 1-inch cubes
1 portobello mushroom, cut in 8 wedges
1 teaspoon paprika (hot or sweet)
1 teaspoon dried basil
Salt and pepper, as desired
Shredded lettuce, stir-fried cabbage, or grated daikon as a serving bed, if desired

In a large skillet or wok, over medium-high heat, stir-fry the beef in the olive and sesame oils and garlic until all the red has disappeared from the meat (approximately 20 minutes).

Add the remaining ingredients and toss well to coat. Continue to stir-fry, stirring constantly, until the green pepper begins to soften but is still crisp.

Serve on a bed of shredded lettuce, stir-fried cabbage, or grated daikon.

Nearly Fried Rice

PREP TIME: 15 minutes

COOK TIME: 9 minutes

SERVINGS: 4

CARBS PER SERVING: 5 grams

What's a Chinese dinner without fried rice? But if you're low-carbing it, you may not be able to afford the luxury of rice. Here's our solution to help satisfy your cravings without spending all your carbs in one place.

4   tablespoons olive oil
1   clove garlic, minced
3   scallions, sliced
1/3 head small cauliflower,
    grated roughly
    (approximately 2 cups)
1/2 teaspoon peeled and finely
    grated fresh ginger root

3   tablespoons soy sauce
1 1/2 cups cooked chicken, beef,
    pork, or shrimp
    in any combination,
    chopped (very fine)
3   eggs, beaten well

Over a medium flame, heat the olive oil in a large skillet or wok. Add the garlic and scallions. Stir-fry for 1 minute. Add the cauliflower and stir-fry for 6 minutes, mixing constantly. Add the ginger root, soy sauce, and cooked meat or shrimp. Stir and cook for 2 minutes.

Push the mixture to one side of pan and scramble the eggs in the empty side until they are cooked but still moist. Combine the eggs and the rest of the mixture in the pan, stirring well. Cook for 1 more minute.

Serve warm or cold.

VARIATIONS

Add 1/2 cup of sliced, cooked, fresh mushrooms, or 1 cup drained and sliced canned mushrooms, along with the eggs.

Silk Road Hot and Sour Soup

PREP TIME: 15 minutes
COOK TIME: 16 minutes

SERVINGS: 4
CARBS PER SERVING: 5 grams

In the Amara Hotel in Singapore, there's an exclusive restaurant that features the Best of China cuisine prepared by chefs from many of the provinces. We figured that was just about as authentic as one could hope for and we were thrilled to secure a reservation. The pungent taste of the Hot and Sour Soup made it our instant favorite. Here's the low-carb version we enjoy whenever we want (and without calling ahead for seating).

1 quart chicken stock (or our Classic Chicken Stock, page 66)
1 chunk fresh ginger root, about 1 inch square, peeled, then thinly sliced
1/2 pound pork loin, cut into 1-inch cubes
2 tablespoons soy sauce
1/4 cup white vinegar
1/2 can (8 ounces) sliced bamboo shoots, drained
1/2 jar (6 1/2 ounces) sliced mushrooms, drained

1/2 block (about 2 × 4 inches) tofu*, drained and cut into 1-inch cubes
1/4 cup chopped daikon
1 teaspoon hot sauce
Ground black pepper, as desired
3 eggs
2 teaspoons arrowroot powder dissolved in 4 teaspoons of water, for thickening (optional)

Heat the chicken stock in a medium-size pot over medium heat. Add the ginger and simmer for 4 minutes. Add the pork, soy sauce, vinegar, bamboo shoots, and mushrooms. Simmer for 10 minutes more, until the pork is cooked through and white.

Add the tofu and daikon. Simmer for 1 minute only. Add the hot sauce. Remove the pan from the heat.

Taste the soup carefully. Add black pepper, as desired.

In a medium-size bowl, whisk or beat the eggs together. Return the pot to the heat. When the soup begins to boil, pour in the beaten eggs

*See page 6 for our Easy but Essential Tofu Tip.

(continued)

in a thin stream over the surface of the soup. Stir well to thicken the soup, then remove it immediately from the heat.

If desired, add the arrowroot and water mixture for more thickening. Stir constantly to make certain the arrowroot mixture is distributed throughout.

Serve warm.

No-Work Moo Shoo Pork

PREP TIME: 11 minutes

COOK TIME: 15 minutes

SERVINGS: 4

CARBS PER SERVING: 3 grams

A delicious standby for when you want an old favorite but not the trouble or the carbs.

1   clove garlic, minced
8   ounces pork loin, julienne
3   tablespoons peanut oil
1   cup green cabbage, shredded
½   cup mushrooms, sliced

2   scallions, thinly sliced, the quantity divided in half
1   cup canned bean sprouts, drained
3   tablespoons soy sauce

In a large skillet or wok, over high heat, stir-fry the garlic and julienne pork in the peanut oil. Continue to stir and cook until all the meat is white and cooked throughout (at least 12 minutes).

Add the cabbage, mushrooms, and half of the scallions and stir-fry for 3 minutes, turning constantly.

Add the bean spouts and soy sauce. Toss and mix thoroughly and remove from heat immediately.

Serve warm (or cold if your kid is not at the table on time!).

Kung Bao Chicken

PREP TIME: 16 minutes
COOK TIME: 20 minutes

SERVINGS: 4
CARBS PER SERVING: 4 grams

We made this dish for our friends, their eight-year-old son, Jordon, and their four-year-old daughter, Amber. The next time we visited them, little Amber asked us to make our "King Kong" meal. The adults were stumped about what she meant and tried every imaginable interpretation. Finally, Jordon figured it out. So that there's no confusion again, here's Amber's favorite Chinese dish.

1 pound chicken breast halves, cut into 1/2-inch cubes
1 egg white, slightly beaten
1 teaspoon soy sauce
1 medium-size onion, diced
1/4 teaspoon ground black pepper
3 tablespoons olive oil
1/2 teaspoon sesame oil
1/2 teaspoon peanut oil

1 clove garlic, minced
1 teaspoon peeled and finely grated fresh ginger root
1/2 green bell pepper, cut into 1-inch cubes
1 cup cauliflower, cut into 1/2-inch pieces
1 cup chicken stock (or our Classic Chicken Stock, page 66) or water

Place the chicken cubes, egg white, soy sauce, diced onion, and black pepper in a large Ziploc bag. Shake the bag well to coat the chicken and then refrigerate the chicken for 1 hour, turning the bag often.

In a large skillet or wok, heat all three oils together until they are hot but not smoking. Add the garlic and ginger. Stir-fry 1 to 2 minutes, until the ginger is softened. Add the chicken and all of the mixture in the Ziploc bag and stir-fry, stirring constantly, until the chicken pieces turn white and are cooked through (about 16 minutes). Add the green pepper, cauliflower, and chicken stock.

Heat the mixture to boiling over a medium flame, then cover and cook for three minutes.

Drain any excess liquid, if desired, before serving the dish warm.

Citrus Salmon

PREP TIME: 12 minutes

COOK TIME: 12 minutes

SERVINGS: 4

CARBS PER SERVING: 4 grams

Succulent and sweet-tasting, without the carbs, this dish can be enjoyed as an appetizer, as a main meal, or cold the next day as a snack.

1 tablespoon olive oil

3 scallions with large bulbs, minced

4 teaspoons lemon juice, divided into two equal parts

2 tablespoons fresh ginger root, peeled and sliced

2 cloves garlic, minced

1 teaspoon crushed red pepper

4 tablespoons sesame oil

1½ tablespoons olive oil

1½ tablespoons white vinegar

1 teaspoon salt

½ teaspoon ground black pepper

4 salmon fillets, 6 ounces each, ½ inch thick

Coat a baking sheet with 1 tablespoon of olive oil. Put aside.

For the paste, combine the scallions, 2 tablespoons lemon juice, the ginger, garlic, red pepper, 1½ tablespoons sesame oil, 1½ tablespoons olive oil, the vinegar, salt, and pepper in a food processor. Process to a smooth paste.

Coat the salmon fillets with the remaining sesame oil on both sides, then transfer the fish, skin side down, to the oiled baking sheet.

Spread the paste on the upper side of each fillet. Cover and refrigerate 2 hours.

Preheat the oven to 375°F.

Bake the salmon steaks, skin side down, until the flesh is opaque throughout, 8 to 12 minutes.

Serve the steaks warm with a sprinkling of the remaining lemon juice.

COMFORT
FOOD

Low-Carb Macaroni and Cheese

PREP TIME: 8 minutes	SERVINGS: 4
COOK TIME: 12 minutes	CARBS PER SERVING: 5 grams

It was our friend Rob's fortieth birthday. He had been counting too many numbers on both the calendar and the scale for his liking, so he had begun a low-carb diet. We surprised him with this treat to remind him that he could stay on his program and still feel like a kid celebrating his own special day.

Cheese Sauce Ingredients

3   teaspoons butter
1   cup light whipping cream
    Salt, black pepper, and
    cayenne pepper, as desired
3/4 cup grated cheese (cheddar,
    American, Swiss, or
    Monterey Jack)

1/2 head cauliflower, florets
    only, cut into individual
    florets
    Any (or all) of the
    following as optional
    garnish: paprika (hot or
    sweet), cayenne, grated
    Parmesan cheese, fresh
    chopped parsley

Preheat the oven 275° F.

In an oven-proof saucepan, prepare the Cheese Sauce portion of our Smooth and Cheesy Crabmeat Casserole recipe (page 253).

Cover and place in the oven to keep warm.

In a medium-size skillet, add water until the level reaches 1 1/2 inches. Turn the heat on high and cover the skillet. When the water reaches full boil, add the cauliflower florets, replace the cover, and cook for 4 minutes.

Remove the skillet from the heat, drain and discard liquid, and transfer the cooked florets to a 2-quart heatproof casserole dish.

Remove the cheese sauce from the oven and pour it over the cooked cauliflower florets. Toss gently to spread the sauce throughout.

Garnish the dish with any one (or all) of the following: paprika, cayenne, grated Parmesan, or fresh chopped parsley.

Classic Chicken Stock

PREP TIME: 15 minutes
COOK TIME: 2½ hours

SERVINGS: 6 to 8 cups stock
CARBS PER SERVING: 2 grams per half cup

Chicken or beef stock is such an essential ingredient in so many low-carb recipes that we make it by the pot. After it has cooled, we freeze it in 2-cup serving sizes in Ziploc freezer bags. Then, when we need it, we just run hot water over the outside of the freezer bag to loosen the frozen stock and drop it out of the bag into a saucepan or microwaveable container. When any meat, chicken, fish, or vegetable recipe needs extra zip, we use this stock instead of water. And, of course, it makes a perfect broth when you're fighting off a nasty cold.

1 (2 pounds) roasting chicken (or fryer), with skin, cut in pieces
4 to 6 cups water
2 bay leaves
2 tablespoons dried basil
2 tablespoons chopped fresh parsley (or 1 tablespoon dried parsley flakes)

3 stalks celery, diced
6 mushrooms, sliced
4 scallions, green part only, diced
4 cloves garlic, minced
   Salt and pepper, as desired

Place the chicken, water, and all other ingredients in a large soup pot or stockpot. Be sure there's enough water to completely cover the chicken.

Cook over medium heat, covered, keeping the liquid at a gentle rolling boil for two hours or until the chicken begins falling off the bone. Allow the stock to cool until it is easily handled.

Remove the bay leaves and all skin and bones. (Double-check this.)

In four separate batches, spoon the stock mixture, along with the chicken meat, into a blender or food processor. Blend each batch of stock well and, after blending, return it to pot.

Simmer the blended stock over medium heat for an additional 30 minutes.

Serve warm.

(continued)

VARIATIONS

Classic Beef Stock: substitute a 2-pound pot roast, cut into 2-inch cubes, for the chicken in the Classic Chicken Stock recipe.

Chinese Chicken/Beef Stock: Add the following ingredients to the Classic Chicken/Beef Stock recipe above and cook in the same way:

1 teaspoon peeled and finely grated fresh ginger root

1 tablespoon chopped coriander stalks

Before cooking, add up to a total of 2 cups (no more than ½ cup each) of any of the following low-carb vegetables: green beans, wax beans, snap beans, green pepper chunks, daikon, bamboo shoots, cauliflower, or additional mushrooms. After cooking, puree in blender and food processor to form a rich stock.

Succulent Salmon with Dill Sauce

PREP TIME: 16 minutes
COOK TIME: 12 minutes

SERVINGS: 4
CARBS PER SERVING: 5 grams

Sometimes your tummy (or your mood) calls for something light. Though subtle, the flavors in this dish blend well. The fish is delicious all by itself. Add the Dill Sauce only if you want some extra pizzazz.

Dill Sauce

1/2 cup sour cream
1 tablespoon scallions, diced
2 tablespoons fresh dill, chopped

1/2 cup mayonnaise
1 tablespoon lemon juice

Succulent Salmon

2 tablespoons butter
2 scallions, chopped
4 salmon fillets, 6 ounces each, 1/2 inch thick
2 cups chicken stock (or our Classic Chicken Stock, page 66)

4 sprigs fresh parsley, chopped (dry equivalent: 1 teaspoon)
1 lemon, cut into thin slices crosswise
Salt and pepper, as desired

Mix the ingredients for the Dill Sauce together well and chill for 1 hour. While the sauce is chilling, prepare the fish.

Melt the butter in a sauté pan or skillet over low heat. Add the scallions and stir until soft, about 2 minutes.

Add the salmon, turn, and cook in butter 1 minute on each side. Pour the chicken stock into the pan.

Simmer over medium heat, covered, for at least 8 minutes (after reaching a boil), until the salmon is cooked throughout.

Remove from the heat. Transfer the fish to a serving platter, discarding the stock. Sprinkle the fish with the parsley, surround with the lemon slices, and season with salt and pepper as desired. Serve the Dill Sauce on the side.

Very Personal Pizza

PREP TIME: 8 minutes
COOK TIME: 12 minutes

SERVINGS: 1
CARBS PER SERVING: 4 grams

In general, how we like our pizza is a personal matter. Each of us prefers certain parts (the crust versus the soggier middle) and particular temperatures (cold for breakfast versus only when hot). This recipe satisfies all requests. Be inventive: add whichever low-carb proteins or veggies you like. It's your diet and your pizza. That's why the recipe is only for one!

1 tablespoon olive oil
1 portobello mushroom, stem removed
1/4 small fresh tomato, blended or processed in a food processor (optional)

2 ounces sausage, fully cooked (or our Freedom Sausage, page 23, fully cooked)
2 ounces mozzarella cheese, cut into 1/4-inch slices
Dash of oregano

Preheat the oven to 400°F.

Brush a baking sheet with some of the olive oil.

Brush the underside of the portobello mushroom with the remaining olive oil and place it, inverted, on the baking sheet.

Layer the processed tomato and sausage over the mushroom, then top with the mozzarella slices. Add a dash of oregano, as desired.

Bake for 12 minutes, or until the cheese begins to bubble (but does not brown).

Gentle Asparagus Purée

PREP TIME: 7 minutes

COOK TIME: 7 minutes

SERVINGS: 2

CARBS PER SERVING: 4 grams

When we're tired or not feeling well, we often don't want anything heavy. That's when this recipe helps us treat ourselves with care.

2 cups water
12 asparagus spears, 3¹/₂-inch lengths from the top
2 tablespoons butter

¹/₄ cup heavy cream
Romano or Parmesan cheese, grated, as desired
Ground black pepper, as desired

In a saucepan, over medium heat, bring the water to a boil. Reduce the heat slightly. Add the asparagus tips and cook at a slow boil for 7 minutes. Drain well.

Transfer to a blender. Add the butter and purée. Add the cream a little at a time, puréeing between each addition until desired consistency is achieved.

Transfer the mixture to individual bowls and stir in cheese and pepper, as desired.

VARIATIONS

Cream of Asparagus Soup: While the asparagus is in the blender, add all the cream and ¹/₄ cup of reserved cooking liquid. Add the butter, cheese, and pepper, and purée. Reheat and serve with a sprinkling of Romano or Parmesan cheese and fresh parsley.

If preferred, substitute cauliflower for asparagus in both purée and soup recipes.

Timeless Quiche

PREP TIME: 15 minutes

COOK TIME: 1 hour

SERVINGS: 4

CARBS PER SERVING: 5 grams

This timeless recipe seems special each time we make it.

Nonstick cooking spray

1½ cups heavy cream

4 slices bacon, cooked crisp and crumbled

1 package (10 ounces) frozen spinach, defrosted and squeezed free of liquid

1 cup grated cheese (cheddar or American)

2 teaspoons finely chopped onion

¼ teaspoon paprika (hot or sweet)

1 teaspoon dried basil

4 eggs

Preheat the oven to 325°F.

Spray a 9-inch pie dish with nonstick cooking spray.

In a medium-size saucepan over a medium flame, stirring constantly, heat the cream, bacon, and spinach until bubbles begin to form around edges. Reduce the heat to low and add the cheese, stirring continuously.

When the cheese is completely melted, add the onion, paprika, and basil.

Remove the pan from the heat and let it cool.

In a small dish, beat the eggs well.

Add one quarter of the beaten egg mixture to the cooled cheese mixture, stirring well after each addition. Beat the egg mixture well before each addition. Stir the cheese mixture well one final time before pouring it into the prepared pie dish.

Bake for about 45 minutes, until custard is set.

Serve warm or cold, as an appetizer or a snack, side dish or main.

Hungarian Creamed Mushrooms

PREP TIME: 8 minutes
COOK TIME: 15 minutes

SERVINGS: 4
CARBS PER SERVING: 3 grams

Richard: *When I was growing up in the Bronx, comfort foods were taken very seriously. Give a youngster the wrong food when he wasn't feeling well and you could upset his stomach or delay his recovery. This recipe, served up on buttered toast, was my favorite. I don't want to think how many times I claimed I wasn't feeling well in order to wheedle a serving or two. By the second or third helping, I'm sure my mother got wise to the charade, but she indulged me anyway.*

2 tablespoons butter
1½ cups sliced mushrooms
½ clove garlic, pressed

½ teaspoon sweet paprika
1½ cups sour cream

In a small saucepan, over a low flame, melt the butter.

Add the mushrooms and garlic and sauté very slowly over low heat until the mushrooms release their liquid, about 10 minutes. Do not cook too quickly or the mushrooms will toughen.

Add the paprika. Stir well. Cover, turn off the heat, and allow the mixture to cool for only 3 minutes.

Add the sour cream by the spoonful, stirring constantly until it is incorporated, and serve.

Hot Spinach Cheese Dip

PREP TIME: 10 minutes

COOK TIME: 30 minutes

SERVINGS: 4

CARBS PER SERVING: 5 grams

We've eaten appetizers with similar names at most of the local restaurant chains, and we think our homemade versions have more flavor than any of them. We cook up three variations on this dish, and when we're eating each one, we swear it's better than the others.

1 tablespoon olive oil

1 cup mayonnaise

1 cup grated cheese (cheddar, American, Swiss, or Monterey Jack)

1/2 cup grated Romano or Parmesan cheese

1 teaspoon minced garlic (or 1/4 teaspoon garlic powder)

1/2 teaspoon black pepper

1/2 teaspoon hot paprika or hot sauce, as desired

1 package (10 ounces) frozen spinach, thawed, drained, and squeezed free of liquid

Low-carb vegetables for dipping

Preheat the oven to 350°F.

Oil a glass 9-inch pie pan, casserole dish, or glass loaf pan. Put it aside.

In a large bowl, combine the mayonnaise, grated cheeses, garlic, black pepper, and paprika or hot sauce as desired. Mix well.

Add the drained spinach and mix well with your hands to ensure complete blending.

Pour the mixture into the pie pan, casserole dish, or loaf pan.

Bake for about 30 minutes, or until dip is heated through and the edges puff (but before the top begins to brown).

Serve hot with low-carb veggies for dipping. Especially good with green pepper slices, celery sticks, and mushroom caps. For a fancier look, serve it up in a green pepper shell.

Sixties Shepherd's Pie

PREP TIME: 15 minutes

COOK TIME: 45 minutes

SERVINGS: 4

CARBS PER SERVING: 4 grams

Shepherd's Pie is a classic comfort food that many of us enjoyed as children. Here's a low-carb version to nourish and comfort you whenever you like.

1 full recipe of Mashed "Potatoes" (without "All the Fixings") (page 210)

1 pound ground beef

1 clove garlic, pressed

1 teaspoon olive oil

6 medium mushrooms, sliced

3 scallions, diced

Salt and pepper

Paprika, hot or sweet, as garnish (optional)

Preheat the oven to 350°F.

Place the full recipe of Mashed "Potatoes" in a medium-size bowl.

In a large nonstick skillet (for maximum contact with the heating surface) over medium-high heat, sauté the ground beef and garlic in no more than 1 teaspoon of olive oil, turning often so that all the meat is browned and cooked through (6 to 8 minutes).

Reduce the heat to medium and add the mushrooms and scallions, continuing to stir until they soften (approximately 3 minutes). Drain off all excess fat.

Remove the skillet from the heat, add salt and pepper as desired, stir, and set aside to cool.

Transfer enough of the cooled meat to just cover the bottom of a 9-inch pie plate. Press down hard. Bake for 5 minutes. Set aside. When cooled, drain all fat and, once again, press down hard to form a meat crust.

Starting with a layer of ground meat (directly on top of the meat crust), alternate between cauliflower Mashed "Potato" mixture and meat layers to form a layered pie, making each layer as thick as you like.

End with a cauliflower Mashed "Potatoes" layer. Sprinkle paprika lightly over the entire top of the pie.

Bake the pie in the oven, uncovered, for 30 minutes.

(continued)

Remove the pie from the oven and cut wedge-shaped slices in it while it's still warm. Allow the pie to cool for a few minutes, then remove the slices carefully from the pan, providing lots of support from underneath. Serve warm or cold.

Soothing Cabbage-Beef Soup

PREP TIME: 15 minutes
COOK TIME: 30 minutes

SERVINGS: 4
CARBS PER SERVING: 4 to 5 grams
(depending on the hot sauce addition)

Served plain or garnished with a slice or two of cheddar cheese, this soothing meal in a bowl will make all of the day's challenges disappear. We make a big pot (three times the recipe) and freeze portions in Ziploc bags. On a moment's notice, we can run a bag under warm water to release the contents, heat up the soup in the microwave or on the stove, and—voilà!—instant warmth.

4 cups chicken stock (or our Classic Chicken Stock, page 66)

2 to 4 cups 1-inch cubes of cooked beef (or cooked pork, chicken, or turkey)

2 cups thinly sliced green cabbage

1/2 small tomato, blended or processed

1 stalk celery, diced

1/2 tablespoon parsley flakes

1/2 tablespoon dried basil

Hot sauce, as desired

Salt and pepper, as desired

2 teaspoons arrowroot powder dissolved in 4 teaspoons of water, for thickening (optional)

2 ounces cheddar cheese, sliced thin (optional)

Place the chicken stock, cooked beef cubes, cabbage, tomato, celery, parsley flakes, basil, and hot sauce, and salt and pepper as desired into a medium-large stock pan. Simmer, covered, over a medium flame in a soft rolling boil for 30 minutes (until the cabbage is soft and tender).

Remove the pan from heat. If desired, add the arrowroot and water mixture for thickening. Stir constantly to make certain the arrowroot mixture is distributed throughout.

If you would like a bubbly cheese topping to your soup, pour individual servings into ovenproof bowls and top with a slice or two of cheddar cheese. Then place the bowls under the broiler for 1 minute, until the cheese melts and turns golden brown.

Serve warm.

(*continued*)

VARIATION

Add 1/2 cup thinly sliced kohlrabi in place of the cabbage for an especially tangy taste.

Great American Cookout
Pork Roast

PREP TIME: 10 minutes

COOK TIME: 2 to 2½ hours

SERVINGS: 8

CARBS PER SERVING: 1 gram

Each Sunday, we spend several hours cooking up a slew of food for the week to come. We put on our favorite CDs or DVDs and whip up several of the recipes in this book, a couple of chickens and steaks, and this pork roast—packing them all away to be used "as needed." We call this our "Great American Cookout." Yet, no matter what we cook, we always end up eating the pork roast that night for dinner. Who said we don't play favorites?

1 (2 pounds) boneless pork roast
1 tablespoon soy sauce
3 tablespoons olive oil
1 tablespoon sesame oil
2 garlic cloves, minced

½ teaspoon ground black pepper
1 teaspoon paprika (hot or sweet)
½ teaspoon Dijon mustard
¼ teaspoon cayenne (optional)

Preheat the oven to 350°F.

Insert a meat thermometer into the thickest part of the pork roast, away from any bones, and set the roast on a rack in a deep baking pan with 1½ inches of water in the bottom of the pan.

In a small screw-top jar, combine the soy sauce and both oils. With the cap on, shake the jar vigorously to mix the ingredients as well as possible, then pour the mixture over all surfaces of the pork, including underneath.

In a small bowl, combine the minced garlic, pepper, paprika, mustard, and cayenne as a rub. Rub it onto all surfaces.

Roast for 2 to 2½ hours, or until the internal temperature reaches 170°F on the meat thermometer.

Add water to the bottom of the roasting pan as needed during the cooking process.

The roast is best sliced after it has cooled for 10 minutes.

Serve warm with au jus gravy formed at the bottom of the pan from the water and meat drippings.

Chill-Fighting Chicken Fricassee

PREP TIME: 15 minutes

COOK TIME: 1 hour

SERVINGS: 4

CARBS PER SERVING: 6 grams

When you're feeling cold and numb from the weather or the stress of the day, this recipe will help warm you up in every way.

1 teaspoon paprika (hot or sweet)
1/2 teaspoon salt
1/4 teaspoon ground black pepper
3 cloves garlic, minced
4 chicken breast halves, boneless and skinless
2 tablespoons unsalted butter

1 1/2 tablespoons chopped onion
1/2 cup chopped celery
2 cups thinly sliced mushroom caps
1 cup Chicken Stock (or our Classic Chicken Stock, page 66)
2 tablespoons chopped fresh parsley, as garnish (optional)

Combine the paprika, salt, pepper, and garlic in a large Ziploc plastic bag. Add the chicken. Toss well to coat the chicken, and then allow it to marinate in the bag in the refrigerator for 1 hour.

Melt the butter in a large nonstick skillet over medium heat. Add the chicken and drippings from the bag, and sauté 5 to 6 minutes, or until the chicken is browned on the outside. (Remember that the chicken is not cooked on the inside yet, so handle it and its juices as if you were dealing with raw chicken. Wash your hands after handling and wash all exposed kitchen and plate surfaces thoroughly with hot soapy water.)

Remove the chicken from the skillet, leaving the drippings in the skillet. Set the chicken aside.

Add the onion, celery, and mushrooms to the pan. Sauté over a moderate flame for 5 minutes, until the onion turns translucent, stirring occasionally. Add the stock and bring to a boil.

Return the chicken to the skillet. Cover, reduce the heat, and simmer for 25 minutes or until the chicken is thoroughly cooked.

Transfer to a serving platter and garnish with chopped parsley.

Kalamata Victory

PREP TIME: 10 minutes

COOK TIME: 1 hour

SERVINGS: 4

CARBS PER SERVING: 4 grams

The olives in this dish get their name from a warrior who started the Revolution of 1821 that freed Greece from four hundred years of Ottoman occupation. If you sometimes feel like you're fighting the whole world, this dish may assure you that all your struggles will have their rewards.

4 chicken breast halves (boneless and skinless), pounded thin	Dash of white vinegar (optional)
2 tablespoons olive oil	1/2 cup crushed pork rinds (optional)
1 teaspoon peanut oil	Wooden toothpicks
1/2 cup drained Kalamata olives, pits removed	

Preheat the oven to 350°F.

In a large skillet over medium heat, brown the pounded chicken breasts in the olive and peanut oils on one side. Flip and brown the other side. Remove the skillet from the heat and drain, setting aside the drippings.

Transfer the chicken to a cool plate.

Place the olives in a blender, add the vinegar and pork rinds, and purée until the olive mixture becomes a paste. Add a few drops of olive oil as needed to achieve desired consistency.

Spread 1 to 2 rounded tablespoons of the olive mixture on the short end of each flattened chicken breast. Roll the chicken and secure it with toothpicks.

Place the rolls onto a cookie sheet and bake, seam side down, for 50 minutes, until cooked through.

Remove the toothpicks and serve warm.

Creamy-Rich Dinner Omelet

PREP TIME: 5 minutes
COOK TIME: 10 minutes

SERVINGS: 2
CARBS PER SERVING: 2 to 5 grams
(depending on choice of additions)

Richard: *When we're facing a long day at work and we know we won't be getting home until late, Rachael will often transfer a package of frozen spinach from the freezer to the refrigerator. That's her way of saying that when we finally do get home, she wants a dinner that she knows can be whipped up in only a few minutes. An important tip: Don't be tempted to make this omelet without sour cream. Its richness makes this dish that much more pleasurable.*

4 large eggs
1 tablespoon milk or cream
2 teaspoons olive oil or butter, divided
1/2 cup frozen spinach, thawed, drained, and squeezed free of liquid

1/2 cup cooked leftovers: meat, poultry, and/or low-carb vegetables
1 teaspoon dried basil (optional)
Salt and pepper, as desired
4 tablespoons sour cream

In a medium-size bowl, combine the eggs and milk/cream. Beat slightly with a fork.

Place one half of the olive oil or butter in a small saucepan, and over a very low flame heat the spinach, cooked leftovers, and basil. Mix well and continue to heat (rather than cook) the mixture, stirring occasionally to keep it from sticking.

Place the remaining olive oil or butter in a medium-large skillet and heat over a medium flame. Pour the egg mixture into the pan and rotate the pan to cover bottom evenly.

As the eggs begin to set, insert a fork at several points and pull gently toward the center of the omelet to allow all of the egg mixture to become exposed to the hot pan.

When completely set (2 to 3 minutes), flip the omelet and cook the other side until it is no longer wet (about 1 minute).

Transfer the heated spinach and leftovers mixture from the small pan to one half of the omelet and spread evenly. Add salt and pepper,

(continued)

as desired, and top with sour cream. Fold the empty side of the omelet over to cover the mixture. Cook for 1 minute.

Flip and cook on the other side until cooked through.

VARIATIONS

We love to add precooked (or canned) mushrooms to this omelet and substitute 2 tablespoons cream cheese for 2 tablespoons of the sour cream. If you use cream cheese, be sure to cook the omelet long enough to melt the cream cheese within the omelet's fold.

Add lox as well as cream cheese and you have a great breakfast or brunch omelet. Follow the first variation above and add a few tablespoons of chopped lox or a strip of lox about 1 inch by 3 inches long. Use nova lox for a less salty omelet.

COOL AND
REFRESHING

Cool Green Pinwheel Salad

PREP TIME: 10 minutes

COOK TIME: none

SERVINGS: 4

CARBS PER SERVING: 2 grams

Simple and quick, this salad is unique in its presentation. A great way to cool off.

1 large cucumber, peeled and diced

6 scallions, green parts only, thinly sliced crosswise

1 large green bell pepper, diced

2 cups alfalfa spouts

8 spinach leaves, washed well and torn

Crisp, crumbled bacon and/or grated cheese of choice (optional)

On a chilled large round serving plate, place the cucumber, scallions, green pepper, and alfalfa sprouts in pinwheel fashion on a bed of torn spinach leaves, so that each pie-shaped quarter contains a different green vegetable. Leave an empty two-inch border around the outer edge of the plate.

Circle the pinwheel with a thin line of bacon bits and/or grated cheese.

Fill in the rest of border with retained torn spinach leaves.

Drizzle with the low-carb salad dressing of your choice (or our Mint Julep Dressing, page 86).

Mint Julep Dressing

PREP TIME: 4 minutes
COOK TIME: none

SERVINGS: 8 (¼ cup each)
CARBS PER SERVING: 2 grams

We first tasted a version of this dressing on our maiden rafting trip on the South Island of New Zealand. It was served at lunch as a dipping sauce alongside piles of fresh raw vegetables. After a morning of hair-raising close calls with disaster on the river, we figured that anything would taste wonderful because we were just happy to be alive. Weeks later, when we whipped up this variation in the safety of our own home, however, we found that it tasted as good as we remembered.

1 cup mayonnaise
1 cup buttermilk

3 tablespoons finely chopped fresh mint leaves
Dash of salt

Combine the ingredients in a large screw-top jar. With the cap on, shake the jar vigorously to mix the dressing well. Refrigerate for at least two hours, shaking every half hour to ensure that the mint flavor infuses the dressing.

Keep refrigerated and shake well before using.

Tangy Olive Nibbles

PREP TIME: 5 minutes

COOK TIME: 5 minutes

SERVINGS: 2 (4 olives each)

CARBS PER SERVING: 2 grams

We expected our first Super Bowl party to be a lot of fun, but we weren't sure how much we'd enjoy watching everyone eat the high-carb goodies . . . for hours. No problem! While everyone else munched enough junk food to feed a small army, we enjoyed these little nuggets with the Polynesian Wings (page 114) we brought as our contribution to the day's potluck dinner. Later, while everyone sat around complaining about their weight and how tired and bloated they felt, we reached for another helping.

5 ounces white vinegar
1/2 cup water
1 clove garlic, pressed
1 teaspoon pickling spice
1 teaspoon dried dill

1/4 teaspoon dried basil
1 can (8 ounces) jumbo pitted whole black ripe olives, drained

In a small saucepan over a low flame, warm the vinegar, water, garlic, pickling spice, dill, and basil. The pickling spice will float on top. Heat the liquid until it is just warm, *not* hot.

Place the olives in a bowl and cover them with the warmed liquid mixture. Marinate, covered, overnight.

Drain and serve ice cold.

Blended Raita Freeze

PREP TIME: 5 minutes   SERVINGS: 4 (¼ cup each)

COOK TIME: none   CARBS PER SERVING: 3 grams

Timing is everything in this recipe. If you make it right, you will find that every hot summer day becomes another excuse to enjoy whipping it up and pouring it over your favorite salad.

½ cucumber, peeled, seeded, and grated

½ cup sour cream

½ cup buttermilk

Dash ground cumin

Place all the ingredients in a blender. Whip at a high speed and pour the contents into 2 ice cube trays. Place in the freezer for about a half hour, until a thin film of ice begins to form on the surfaces only. Do not allow the mixture to freeze into solid cubes. Check often. The freezing time varies depending on the temperature of your freezer.

Put the contents into a chilled serving pitcher, such as a ceramic or glass creamer, and pour over your favorite salad.

Nova Scotia Salmon Pâté

PREP TIME: 15 minutes

COOK TIME: 5 minutes

SERVINGS: 4

CARBS PER SERVING: 4 grams

One of the most beautiful places in the world is Nova Scotia in the summer. The grass is the greenest, the shoreline the most chiseled, the pine trees the most fragrant, and the sky the bluest we have ever seen. In our little hotel, a pâté was served at breakfast every day, made with fresh salmon caught each morning by the owner. Since we have no intention of getting up before dawn to go fishing, we created this version using canned salmon and enjoy it on hot summer days as a cool way to get our protein.

1 clove garlic, pressed
2 teaspoons green bell pepper, finely diced
4 teaspoons onion, chopped
2 tablespoons butter
3 ounces cream cheese, cubed and softened

1 can (7.5 ounces) red salmon in oil, drained
1 teaspoon fresh parsley, chopped
1/2 tablespoon lemon zest
Salt and pepper, as desired
Raw low-carb vegetables, for serving

In a small skillet over medium heat, sauté the garlic, green pepper, and onion in butter until the green pepper softens and the onion turns translucent (about 5 minutes). Remove from the heat.

Combine the cream cheese, salmon, parsley, lemon zest, and salt and pepper as desired in a food processor or blender. Add the sautéed mixture and process until smooth and well blended.

Transfer the mixture to a small bowl, cover, and chill.

Serve the pâté with celery sticks, green pepper strips, cucumber coins, raw mushroom caps, green beans, snap beans, wax beans, or other low-carb veggies of your choice.

VARIATIONS

Serve the pâté in a green bell pepper or tomato shell.

Double the amount of cream cheese and use the pâté as a stuffing for mushroom caps or celery.

Mound the pâté on an inverted raw portobello mushroom cap and slice the mushroom cap into wedges.

Harvard Mushroom Morsels

PREP TIME: 15 minutes

COOK TIME: 10 minutes

SERVINGS: 4 (3 mushrooms each)

CARBS PER SERVING: 2 grams

The day was gray and the temperature in the teens. Our friends were visiting their oldest son at the Ivy League school he was attending and we promised we would join them. We were greeted by the son's big smile, a shared apartment three times more littered than his room at home, a long list of complaints about the demands of schoolwork and the competitiveness of his peers, and these hors d'oeuvres he had made himself. Well, we concluded, at least he had learned something.

Nonstick cooking spray

12 large mushroom caps, for stuffing

1 tablespoon olive oil

1/4 cup chopped onions

4 ounces ricotta cheese

1/4 cup grated Swiss cheese

1 tablespoon capers

1/2 teaspoon dried basil

Salt and pepper, as desired

Dash hot sauce (optional)

Fresh parsley as garnish (optional)

Preheat the broiler.

Lightly coat a baking sheet with nonstick cooking spray. Place the mushroom caps, inverted, on the sheet so that they are not touching. Set aside.

In a medium-size nonstick skillet, heat the olive oil for 2 minutes, tilting the pan to coat the bottom.

Add the onions and sauté, stirring often to prevent sticking. Cook until the onions have turned golden and begun to crisp. Remove the skillet from the heat, drain the onions with a slotted spatula, and allow them to cool.

In a large bowl, combine the remaining ingredients and the cooled onion. Mix well.

Spoon the mixture into the inverted mushroom caps and broil for 2 minutes, until cheeses are warm and bubbly. Watch carefully to prevent burning.

Remove the mushrooms from the oven and allow them to cool to desired temperature before serving. Garnish with parsley.

Daintree Marinade

PREP TIME: 15 minutes
COOK TIME: 5 minutes

SERVINGS: 4
CARBS PER SERVING: 1 gram

This recipe was born of necessity. We had been offered the opportunity to visit the Daintree Rainforest, the world-famous rainforest in Australia, but we had to leave at that very moment—with no time to buy or prepare any low-carb food. The food the guide brought was (of course!) nothing but carbs. We usually travel with at least two cans of tuna, but after a long day's trek, that didn't quite meet the needs of our growling stomachs. Using all the condiments available to us, we made the grandfather of this recipe on the spot. It has gone through several variations since then, until now we've found the perfect balance.

3/4 cauliflower head
     water
1/2 cup white vinegar
  2 teaspoons Dijon mustard
1/4 teaspoon salt
1/8 teaspoon ground black
     pepper

1/2 teaspoon hot sauce
     (optional)
1/2 cup chopped celery
  1 cup olive oil
     Lettuce leaves (any variety,
     including arugula)
  2 cans (6 ounces each) tuna in
     water, drained

In a medium-size saucepan, add the cauliflower to 2 inches of water. Heat over a high heat and boil for 5 minutes.

Plunge the cauliflower into cold water, to stop cooking, and drain well. Set it aside to cool.

In a small saucepan, over very low heat, combine the vinegar, mustard, salt, pepper, hot sauce, and celery. Warm the mixture only; do not cook. Remove it from the heat. Using a whisk or fork, gradually beat in the oil until well combined. Set aside.

Break the cauliflower into florets and cut the tough inner core of the head into bite-size pieces. Place the florets and pieces in a medium-size shallow bowl.

Pour the vinegar mixture over the cauliflower so that most of the surface area is covered.

(continued)

Cover and refrigerate for 6 to 8 hours or overnight, mixing as often as possible to ensure even coverage with marinade.

Drain the cauliflower well before serving ice cold on a bed of lettuce or arugula, surrounded by a ring of drained canned tuna flakes.

Porcupine Cheese Ball

PREP TIME: 15 minutes
COOK TIME: none

SERVINGS: 3 (½ cup each)
CARBS PER SERVING: 1 gram

Our neighbors called to find out how late we'd be for their six-year-old daughter's birthday celebration and to remind us not to forget the special "party food" we had promised to bring. Birthday party? Food? We'd forgotten all about it! This dish seemed to come together by itself. Some of us work best under pressure.

1 cup grated cheese (cheddar or American)
3 ounces cream cheese, quartered and softened
¼ cup chopped fresh celery leaves
1 tablespoon mayonnaise
¼ teaspoon white prepared horseradish
¼ teaspoon Dijon mustard
¼ teaspoon onion or garlic powder
¼ teaspoon paprika (hot or sweet)
Dash hot sauce (optional)
½ cup crushed pork rinds
3 stalks celery, cut into 3-inch-long sticks

In a large bowl, combine the grated cheese, cream cheese, celery leaves, mayonnaise, horseradish, mustard, onion or garlic powder, paprika, and hot sauce. Shape into a large ball.

Roll the ball in the crushed pork rinds to coat. Insert the celery sticks into the cheese ball, spacing them evenly to approximate porcupine quills.

If time permits, place the ball in a large deep bowl, cover with plastic wrap, and refrigerate for 2 hours. Remove the ball from the refrigerator, place it on a flat plate, and wait about 5 minutes before serving.

Use celery sticks to scoop up excess creamy cheese mixture.

Truly Low-Carb Wraps

PREP TIME: 5 minutes

COOK TIME: 5 minutes

SERVINGS: makes 6 (3½-inch) crepes

CARBS PER SERVING: 0

Some commercially available "low-carb" breads and wraps aren't low-carb at all. For breakfast, lunch, or dinner—or any time in between—this truly low-carb wrap is ready in a few minutes and can open up a world of choices.

2 eggs	4 tablespoons butter
¼ teaspoon cream of tartar	Tuna, chicken, low-carb
2 tablespoons small-curd cottage cheese	meat salads, cottage and cream cheese mixtures, cold
1 tablespoon sour cream	or warm low-carb stir-fry
Choice of cinnamon, rosemary, paprika, dried basil, garlic powder, or onion flakes	dishes, for filling as desired

Separate the whites from the yolks of the eggs. With an electric mixer, beat the egg whites with the cream of tartar until the whites form stiff peaks. Set them aside.

In a medium-size bowl, combine the yolks and cottage cheese. Beat them well with a fork. Add the sour cream and a spice of your choice. Beat well with a fork.

Gently fold the mixture into the egg whites. Stir gently with a spoon until white and yellow mixtures combine.

Melt 2 tablespoons of butter in a nonstick frying pan or griddle over a medium flame.

Drop about 2 tablespoons of the egg batter into the heated pan to form a 3½-inch crepe. Flatten with the rounded part of the tablespoon. Repeat until you've created three crepes. Cook over moderate heat until the crepes are set and appear to be very brown on the bottom (3 to 4 minutes). Turn and brown the other side (about 3 minutes). Continue making crepes until all the batter has been used.

Remove the crepes to a plate and allow them to cool. They will be fluffy but will flatten as they cool. Spread a low-carb filling of your choice down the middle of the crepe and fold over each side to cover

(continued)

the middle. Ice-cold tuna, chicken, low-carb meat salads, cottage and cream cheese mixtures, and cold or warm low-carb stir-fry dishes make excellent fillings.

Serve immediately.

VARIATION

For a low-carb taco, fill the crepe with ground meat, grated cheese, sour cream, and shredded lettuce or our Chili Beef and Cheese dish (page 157).

Sorrel Bisque

PREP TIME: 8 minutes

COOK TIME: 5 minutes

SERVINGS: 6 (½ cup each)

CARBS PER SERVING: 2 grams

Richard: *My mother used to make this wonderful cold soup from an old Hungarian recipe handed down from her grandmother. When my mother passed away, we found a hundred recipes, all in a language I could not read. Rachael and I located a young college student to translate, and this is one of our rewards. We hope you enjoy it as much as we do.*

1 teaspoon butter
¼ pound sorrel (sour grass), washed, dried, and finely chopped
   or
¼ pound fresh spinach (about ⅓ of a bunch), washed, dried, and finely chopped

2 cups chicken broth (or our Classic Chicken Stock, page 66)
4 egg yolks
1 cup heavy cream
   Ground black pepper, as desired

Melt the butter in a medium-size saucepan over a low-medium flame.

Add the sorrel or spinach and sauté in the butter until wilted. Remove from the fire and set aside.

Heat the broth in a small saucepan, not allowing it to boil.

Combine the egg yolks and cream in a small bowl. Mix briskly with a whisk. Stirring constantly, add the egg mixture to the stock while continuing to heat. Do not allow the mixture to boil.

Remove the stock from the heat, add the sorrel or spinach, and mix (the sorrel or spinach may float). Allow the mixture to cool.

Top the bisque with black pepper, as desired, and refrigerate until cold.

Green Salsa

PREP TIME: 12 minutes

COOK TIME: none

SERVINGS: 1½ cup (2 servings)

CARBS PER SERVING: 2 grams

St. Paddy's Day in Dublin—what an experience! The only things that weren't green were some of the faces around us. Friends took us to three pubs in as many hours. The first two had absolutely no low-carb food, and we were not happy. The third pub saved our lives with a great salsa they called "green dipper." Here's our version.

½ cup chopped fresh spinach (or ¼ cup frozen chopped spinach, thawed, drained, and squeezed free of liquid)

1 teaspoon Dijon mustard

1 tablespoon chopped fresh parsley

1 tablespoon chopped scallions

½ green bell pepper, diced finely

3 tablespoons white vinegar

¼ cup olive oil

Salt and pepper, as desired

In a food processor, combine all the ingredients. Process well.

Refrigerate the mixture until it's thoroughly chilled. Serve the salsa as a dip for vegetables, or spoon it over cold leftover cooked meat, fowl, or fish.

VARIATION

Use sour cream instead of olive oil and vinegar. Lighter green, still great taste.

Lemon Zest Chicken Salad

PREP TIME: 15 minutes	**SERVINGS:** 4
COOK TIME: none	**CARBS PER SERVING:** 2 grams

Richard: *As a kid, I was rarely home on time for Saturday lunch and eventually my mother gave up making me a hot meal. This dish worked instead. Sometimes she substituted beef, pork, or turkey for the chicken. I was fifteen before I realized she was using this recipe as an excuse to get rid of Friday night's leftovers. No matter—I loved it then and I still do today.*

1/4 cup mayonnaise
1/4 cup sour cream
1 teaspoon Dijon mustard
2 cups diced cooked chicken
(or beef, pork, or turkey)
1/2 cup crumbled blue cheese
1/4 cup grated cheese (cheddar
or American)

1/4 cup diced scallions
1/2 cup diced celery
1 tablespoon lemon zest
Salt and pepper, as desired
4 to 6 romaine lettuce leaves
2 eggs, hard-boiled, peeled,
and sliced

Combine the mayonnaise, sour cream, and mustard in a large bowl. Stir well.

Slowly add the cooked chicken, blue cheese, grated cheese, scallions, celery, lemon zest, and salt and pepper as desired, tossing well to make certain all the vegetables are thoroughly coated.

Turn the mixture onto a bed of romaine lettuce leaves and circle it with hard-boiled egg slices. Or use the mixture as a satisfying filling in a Truly Low-Carb Wrap (page 94).

VARIATION

Arugula leaves, in place of romaine lettuce, add a lovely peppery flavor to this dish.

Creamy Tuna Tidbits

PREP TIME: 10 minutes
COOK TIME: none

SERVINGS: 2 (4 halves each)
CARBS PER SERVING: 2 grams

Rachael: *This is the perfect Saturday summer lunch for me. Add some green pepper and cucumber slices, a couple of celery sticks, and a glass of iced tea and I'm a happy camper.*

4   hard-boiled eggs, peeled and halved
10 black ripe olives, drained, pitted, and sliced
1/4 cup canned tuna in water, drained and flaked
1   tablespoon mayonnaise

1/4 teaspoon paprika (hot or sweet)
1/4 teaspoon lemon juice
1/4 teaspoon soy sauce
    Salt and pepper, as desired
    Cucumber slices
    Romaine lettuce leaves

Remove the yolks of the hard-boiled eggs and transfer them to a small bowl.

Arrange the egg-white halves on a cake cooling rack. Place the rack over a large serving plate or a surface covered with paper toweling to catch any spills during the stuffing of the egg whites.

Line the cavity of each egg-white half with olive slices. Set aside the remaining olive slices.

Mash the egg yolks, then combine them with the tuna, mayonnaise, paprika, and lemon juice. Add the soy sauce, and salt and pepper as desired. Mix very well.

Spoon the yolk mixture into the cavities of the egg whites. Dot the filled center of each egg-white half with an olive slice or two.

Spread the leftover yolk mixture on cucumber slices. Top the cucumber with sliced olives.

Arrange the egg halves and cucumber slices on a bed of romaine lettuce leaves and serve chilled.

CRUNCHY SATISFACTION

Tofu Crisps

PREP TIME: 3 minutes

COOK TIME: 8 minutes

SERVINGS: 2 (10 crackers each)

CARBS PER SERVING: 1 gram

Once you've tasted these crisps, you'll always want to have them around. They are excellent with salads, dips, and soups, or in place of crackers or bread, and can be whipped up whenever you want them.

1 block (about 4 × 4 inches)   ¼ cup olive oil
firm tofu, drained

Drain the tofu according to our Easy but Essential Tofu Tip (page 6). Place the tofu block on a clean plate or cutting board. Slice once down the center of the tofu from top to bottom to form two bars, 2 × 4 inches each.

Cut each block into thin slices, ¼ inch thick, approximately 1 inch wide and 2 inches long. Repeat this process with the second bar of tofu. Drain excess liquid.

In a large nonstick skillet, over a medium flame, heat the oil until warm.

Carefully transfer the tofu rectangles to the oil (be careful, they will sputter), making one layer, with room between rectangles to allow for turning.

When the edges of the rectangles appear well browned (about 5 minutes), turn them carefully with a spatula.

Cook the tofu until the second side is dark golden brown (another 3 minutes).

Remove the slices to a dry plate and allow them to cool undisturbed.

Serve the crisps with any creamy low-carb dip (or our Four-Spice Creamy Dip, page 273) or hot sauce (or one of our three homemade hot sauces on pages 259, 260, and 261), or enjoy them all by themselves.

Crisp and Crackly
Cheese Crackers

PREP TIME: 1 to 5 minutes

COOK TIME: 6 minutes

SERVINGS: 8 crackers

CARBS PER SERVING: 1 gram

The only problem with these little bits of pleasure is that everyone loves them, including those not on low-carb diets. These crackers disappear so fast, we have to hide them or there won't be any left for us.

8 slices cheese (Use cheddar, Colby, or Swiss cheese *only*), sliced medium. (Note: If you're using Swiss cheese, remove and discard the rind prior to heating.)

Heat a nonstick pan over medium-high heat. Lay the cheese slices on the bottom of the pan so that they do not touch.

Allow them to cook, without touching, for approximately 3 minutes. The cheese will begin to bubble, forming holes. Clear oil will run off and the cheese will begin to turn golden.

With a nonstick spatula (with a thin edge on its plastic blade), tease up the edges of the cheese so that you can see the underside of the slices. When the underside of the cheese is light golden brown, start carefully teasing up the edges until you can pick the slices up and turn them over.

The second side will cook more quickly. When it is golden, lift the cheese with a spatula onto a plate lined with paper towels. Do not turn the slices over.

For crackers, allow the slices to cool completely and break each slice into quarters. To form a crackly bowl ideal for cold salads and other lightweight foods, lay a still-warm cheese slice fresh from the pan over a small overturned bowl. When the cheese is cool enough to touch, gently push in on the sides to conform the cheese to the shape of the bowl. Allow it to cool completely, then very carefully remove it from the bowl.

Waldorf Lamb Salad

PREP TIME: 15 minutes

COOK TIME: none

SERVINGS: 4

CARBS PER SERVING: 2 grams

The first time we visited the Undara Lava Tubes in Australia, we went by horseback. When we stopped for lunch, our guide served us a salad straight out of the cooler. If the Lava Tubes hadn't been so breathtaking and the meal so crunchy and refreshing, we would have turned back after half a day. By the end of the second day of nonstop horseback riding, we sorely wished we had. Here's our re-creation of that much appreciated salad.

1/2 cup sour cream
1/2 cup mayonnaise
 1 teaspoon Dijon mustard
1/2 cup 1-inch cubes of daikon
1/4 cup pitted, sliced olives
   (green olives or black ripe,
   drained)

 2 cups diced cooked lamb (or
   shrimp, chicken, turkey,
   or beef)
1/2 cup grated Colby cheese
1/4 cup diced scallions
 1 tablespoon lime zest
1/2 tablespoon lime juice
   Salt, pepper, and hot sauce,
   as desired

In a large bowl, combine the sour cream, mayonnaise, and mustard. Stir well.

Add all the remaining ingredients, tossing to make sure each ingredient is coated well.

Refrigerate and serve cold.

VARIATIONS

Serve the salad with Crisp and Crackly Cheese Crackers or in a Crisp-and-Crackly-Cheese-Cracker bowl (page 104).

Spoon the finished salad into Truly Low-Carb Wraps (page 94).

BLT Snack Pockets

PREP TIME: 5 minutes
COOK TIME: none

SERVINGS: 2
CARBS PER SERVING: 2 grams

We love old-fashioned bacon, lettuce, and tomato sandwiches. This low-carb version has stood the test of time: we've been enjoying these pockets for two decades. Vary the low-carb dressing and the pockets take on a whole new flavor. Add hard-boiled egg slices and you have a great breakfast treat.

4 large romaine leaves, washed and patted dry
6 slices bacon, cooked crisp and chopped
1/4 cup diced tomato
1/2 cup finely shredded lettuce (any variety)
1/4 cup diced cucumber

1/4 cup diced celery
8 black ripe olives, drained, pitted, and sliced (optional)
Your favorite low-carb salad dressing (or our Mint Julep Dressing, page 86) or mayonnaise

Cut off the tough bottom half of the romaine leaves and discard them. Then trim the softer top half into rectangles. Set aside.

In a large mixing bowl, toss the bacon, tomato, lettuce, cucumber, celery, and olive slices. Drizzle with salad dressing and mix thoroughly.

Place 2 to 3 tablespoons of the salad mixture in the center of each large romaine leaf.

Fold from the two sides toward the center, then top and bottom toward the center, overlapping, to form a pocket.

VARIATIONS

Serve with Crisp and Crackly Cheese Crackers (page 104).

In place of lettuce leaves as pockets, spoon the finished salad mixture into Truly Low-Carb Taco Wraps (page 95).

Before folding in the lettuce sides, top the salad mixture with a slice or two of hard-boiled egg and you have an easy, delicious, crunchy breakfast delight.

For a crunchy, fresh-tasting addition, top the salad mixture with a layer of alfalfa sprouts before folding the leaf into a pocket.

Chicken Medallions

PREP TIME: 15 minutes

COOK TIME: 40 minutes

SERVINGS: 4 (6 medallions each)

CARBS PER SERVING: 3 grams

Pop a couple of these into your mouth when you're aching for a snack. Better yet, dip them in our Instant Onion Dip (page 225) or our Big Jim's Blood-in-Your-Eye Barbecue Sauce (page 19), add some ice-cold celery sticks and a cup of warm coffee or tea, and you've got a meal that will leave you with a smile on your face.

2 chicken breast halves, pounded thin
1/2 pound mozzarella cheese, thinly sliced
8 strips bacon, cooked crisp and drained

2 teaspoons minced fresh garlic (or 1/2 teaspoon garlic powder)
2 teaspoons soy sauce
2 tablespoons olive oil

Preheat the oven to 350°F.

Place one pounded chicken breast flat on an oiled baking sheet, so that it is longer than it is wide.

Lay the slices of mozzarella over the chicken. Lay 4 strips of bacon evenly across the width of the chicken breast (from side to side). Sprinkle each chicken breast with half the garlic, soy sauce, and olive oil.

Roll the breasts up, jelly-roll style, starting from the bottom, to form a log.

Place them seam side down on a baking sheet.

Bake for 40 minutes or until golden brown.

Remove from the oven and allow the breasts to cool while still on the baking sheet, then refrigerate for 2 hours.

Slice each log into 1/2-inch coins, which can be enjoyed with your favorite low-carb dipping sauce or Dijon mustard.

For extra crunch, immediately before eating, fry each coin for 2 minutes on each side in 1/4 inch of hot olive oil, then drain on a paper towel and allow to cool on a dry plate.

Salmon Croquettes

PREP TIME: 7 minutes

COOK TIME: 9 minutes

SERVINGS: 2 (2 patties each)

CARBS PER SERVING: 2 grams

Rachael: *This was the first dinner I ever made. My father and I were eating at home alone and I was suddenly the "lady of the house." At ten, I was very proud of my achievement and made him eat patty after patty to prove he liked them.*

2 cans (7.5 ounces) red salmon, drained, large bones and skin removed

2 eggs, beaten well

1 cup crushed pork rinds

1 teaspoon parsley flakes

1/2 teaspoon dried basil

1/4 cup minced onion

1 1/2 teaspoons lemon juice

1/8 teaspoon ground black pepper

2 to 3 tablespoons olive oil

In a large mixing bowl, combine the salmon, eggs, pork rinds, parsley, basil, onion, lemon juice, and black pepper. Mix very well with your hands, crushing the salmon chunks into the mixture.

Shape the mixture into patties about 3 inches in diameter.

In a large nonstick skillet, over a medium flame, heat the olive oil. Place the patties one by one in the hot oil, leaving enough room between them to manipulate a spatula for turning.

Gently, with a nonstick spatula, lift the patties to view the underside. When the underside is golden brown and the inside is hot enough so that the egg has cooked (about 5 minutes), support the top of the patty and flip it over.

Fry until golden brown on the other side (3 to 4 minutes).

North Queensland Greek Salad

PREP TIME: 15 minutes

COOK TIME: none

SERVINGS: 2

CARBS PER SERVING: 3 grams

Yanni's Restaurant in Cairns, Australia, serves the crispest Greek salad in the world. We've asked them a thousand times why their vegetables are so crunchy. "Ahh," says handsome Yanni, with a flash of white teeth against his tan face. "Those are the secrets that make us the best!" We suspect they soak some of their vegetables in ice water just long enough to bring out the crunchiness. Here's our low-carb adaptation.

4 cups crisp lettuce leaves (romaine or iceberg), torn into salad-size pieces

1 medium cucumber, peeled and chopped

1/2 green bell pepper, cored, seeded, and cut into 1-inch cubes

4 ounces feta cheese, crumbled

4 ounces Greek black olives, pits removed

Dressing

2 tablespoons olive oil

2 teaspoons lemon juice

1/2 tablespoon dried oregano

1 teaspoon crushed garlic

Salt and pepper, as desired

Tear the lettuce leaves into salad-size pieces (2- to 3-inch squares) and place them in a large salad bowl. Combine all the remaining salad ingredients and toss lightly.

Place the dressing ingredients in a small screw-top jar. Secure the cover and shake the jar well.

Drizzle the dressing liberally on the salad and toss well.

Serve immediately or refrigerate the salad, covered, for 1 hour and serve ice cold.

Cracklin' Duck

We save this dish for our most special occasions. The secret to the crunch is in basting the duck often and cooking it at just the right temperature to ensure that the duck skin is the crispiest it can be without burning.

Marinade

4 cups chicken stock (or our Classic Chicken Stock, p. 66)

2 teaspoons lime juice

2 teaspoons soy sauce

1 teaspoon dried basil

1/2 teaspoon sage

1/2 cup chopped watercress or chopped parsley

1/2 cup chopped celery

Salt, ground black pepper, and hot sauce, as desired

1 small duckling (2 to 2 1/2 pounds), quartered

Glaze

1/2 cup peanut or sesame oil

1/3 cup olive oil

6 tablespoons lime zest

Combine all the marinade ingredients in a large stockpot. Heat the mixture over a medium flame until it is just warm (not hot). Allow the marinade to cool completely.

Add the duck quarters and allow them to marinate, covered, in the refrigerator, for 2 to 4 hours.

Meanwhile, combine the ingredients for the glaze in a medium-size bowl and allow the mixture to sit at room temperature while the duck marinates.

When the marinating time is up, remove the duck quarters from the marinade, drain them, and dry them with paper towels.

Preheat the oven to 400°F.

(continued)

Place the duck quarters on a rack in a shallow roasting pan in which there is 1 inch of water.

Spoon ⅓ of the glaze over the duck quarters, making certain that any glaze that comes in contact with the duck drips into the water in the bottom of the roasting pan and does *not* drip back into the unused glaze.

Baste twice more as above while maintaining 1 inch of water in the bottom of the roasting pan (below the rack).

Roast the duck on the rack for 40 minutes, until cooked through.

Serve warm with au jus gravy from the bottom of the pan.

Shrimp and Bacon Bowl

PREP TIME: 12 minutes

COOK TIME: 5 minutes

SERVINGS: 4

CARBS PER SERVING: 5 grams

Make it once, enjoy it twice . . . warm now and cold tomorrow.

3 tablespoons olive oil
1 tablespoon peanut oil
1 tablespoon crushed garlic
1 tablespoon dried basil
1 tablespoon dried tarragon
1 teaspoon lime zest
1 pound medium raw shrimp, cleaned, shelled, and deveined
1 teaspoon lemon juice

1 tablespoon chopped scallions
1 cup diced daikon
1/2 cup diced celery
Salt and pepper, as desired
4 slices bacon, cooked crisp, chopped
4 green bell peppers, cored and seeded, ice cold
Paprika or fresh parsley as garnish (optional)

Combine the oils, garlic, basil, tarragon, and lime zest in a large skillet and heat over a medium-high flame until hot. (Alternatively, heat a wok until a few beads of water dripped from your fingertips dance and evaporate on contact. Add the oils and tilt the wok to coat the inside surface. Continue to heat the oils for an additional 20 seconds, then add the garlic, basil, tarragon, and lime zest, stirring continuously.)

Add the shrimp and stir continuously, making certain that all sides of the shrimp make contact with the hot surfaces of the skillet (or wok). Cook for 2 minutes.

Add the lemon juice, scallions, daikon, celery, and salt and pepper as desired, and continue to stir-fry without stopping for an additional 2 minutes. The dish is ready when the shrimp flesh is white and thoroughly cooked. Remove it from the heat, add the bacon pieces, and stir well.

Remove the green pepper shells from the refrigerator and fill the cavities with the shrimp mixture.

Garnish with paprika or fresh parsley and serve warm, or for maximum crunch, refrigerate until ice cold.

(continued)

VARIATIONS

If you prefer a warm green pepper shell, steam the shells in a deep saucepan over a medium-high flame in 1¹/₂ inches of water, covered, for 5 minutes.

Substitute romaine lettuce leaves for green pepper if desired (1 gram of carbs less per serving). Fold the leaves as described for our BLT Snack Pockets (page 106).

Polynesian Wings

PREP TIME: 6 minutes

COOK TIME: 40 to 50 minutes

SERVINGS: 4

CARBS PER SERVING: 1 gram

The chefs at the Polynesian Hotel at Disney World put tang and crunch into all of their signature dishes, and as an unexpected bonus, many of the dishes are naturally low in carbs. Here's our own variation of a great dish (one of many) we have enjoyed often at their Kona Kafe.

5 tablespoons olive oil
1/2 cup lemon juice
2 to 4 tablespoons soy sauce
2 to 4 tablespoons Dijon mustard

2 pounds chicken or turkey wings, rinsed and dried with paper towels
2 teaspoons paprika (hot or sweet)
2 teaspoons garlic powder

Preheat the oven to 350°F.

Oil two baking sheets, using one tablespoon of the olive oil.

Place the lemon juice in a large, shallow bowl.

In a second large, shallow bowl, combine the remaining olive oil, the soy sauce, and the mustard. Mix well.

Using your hands, first dip each wing into the lemon juice, then smear it thickly with the soy-mustard mixture. Make a second batch of soy mixture as needed.

Arrange the wings at equal distances on the baking sheets. Sprinkle them well with paprika and garlic powder.

Bake for 40 to 45 minutes for chicken wings or 50 minutes for turkey wings, until thoroughly cooked. The outside skin should be browned and very crunchy, and the meat should not be pink at all, even at the joints.

Crunchy Vegetable-Beef Soup

PREP TIME: 20 minutes

COOK TIME: 45 minutes

SERVINGS: 6 (1 cup each)

CARBS PER SERVING: 2 grams

We can always judge how fresh the food is at a restaurant by sampling the vegetable soup. Mushy vegetables? The chef is getting rid of old leftovers or keeping the soup hot all day so he doesn't have to take the trouble of individually preparing your meal. Crunchy vegetables? The chef cares about his customers and your dining experience.

1 tablespoon olive oil

1 tablespoon butter

2 cloves garlic, crushed

1/4 cup chopped onion

1/2 pound sirloin or strip steak, cut into 1-inch cubes

4 cups beef broth (or our Classic Beef Stock, page 67)

1/2 tomato, diced

1/2 cup coarsely chopped cauliflower

1 stalk celery, chopped

1/2 cup chopped green bell peppers

3 large mushroom caps, sliced

1/2 cup 3/4-inch cubes of daikon (optional)

2 1/2 tablespoons chopped fresh parsley

1/3 teaspoon dried oregano

1 tablespoon dried basil

Salt, pepper, and hot sauce, as desired

2 teaspoons arrowroot powder dissolved in 4 teaspoons of water, for thickening (optional)

Grated Parmesan cheese

In a very large nonstick skillet, combine the olive oil and butter and heat over a medium flame until the butter has melted and the oil is hot (but not smoking).

Add the garlic and onion and stir. Cook until the onion turns brown and crispy, stirring often.

Add the steak cubes and stir, constantly exposing all surfaces of the meat to the hot oil and hot pan. Continue to cook and stir for a total of 7 minutes. Remove the skillet from the heat.

Transfer the meat and some of the drippings to a large stockpot. Add the beef stock and cook, partially covered, over a medium-high flame at a gentle rolling boil for 30 minutes.

While the meat and broth cook, place the tomato, cauliflower, celery, green peppers, and mushroom caps into the meat skillet, which

(continued)

still contains some drippings. Cook over a medium-high flame, stirring constantly, for 3 minutes. Remove the skillet from the heat. Stir the mixture and allow it to cool slightly. Add the vegetable mixture to the beef and stock, and cook for another five minutes.

When the meat and broth have cooked for a full 30 minutes and the vegetables have been in the stock for only 5 minutes, remove the pot from the heat. Immediately add the daikon, parsley, oregano, basil, and salt and pepper and hot sauce as desired to the soup pot and stir well.

If desired, add the arrowroot and water mixture for thickening. Stir constantly to make certain the arrowroot mixture is distributed throughout.

Allow the soup to cool to your ideal temperature for eating. Transfer it to individual bowls, top with grated Parmesan, and serve.

New Orleans Blackened Tuna

PREP TIME: 10 minutes

COOK TIME: 9 minutes

SERVINGS: 4

CARBS PER SERVING: 1 gram

We were in New Orleans at our first scientific meeting together, presenting the results of two long years of research. We only had enough money for one good meal but there were four days of eating to pay for. For three days, we shared a salad bowl at our local fast-food restaurant. After our presentation was accepted with cheers, we went to the seafood restaurant that had beckoned us since our arrival and splurged on a victory meal, the inspiration for this dish.

1 teaspoon salt	1/2 teaspoon dried thyme
1/2 teaspoon ground black pepper	1/2 teaspoon dried oregano
1 tablespoon paprika (hot or sweet)	1 tablespoon dried basil
1/2 teaspoon cayenne pepper, as desired	1/2 teaspoon dried tarragon (optional)
1 teaspoon onion flakes	3/4 cup butter
1 teaspoon garlic powder	2 tablespoons olive oil
	2 pounds tuna fillets (4 fillets, 1/2 to 3/4 inch thick)

In a small bowl or Ziploc plastic bag, mix the dry ingredients well. Transfer the mixture to a large plate.

In a heavy skillet (do *not* use a nonstick or lightweight skillet), over medium heat, melt the butter. Transfer it to a wide, shallow bowl.

Place the olive oil in the same heavy skillet, tilting to completely cover the bottom.

Turn on a hood vent or open a window and turn the heat under the skillet to high.

Dip each tuna fillet in the melted butter, then dip it in the dry mixture, patting the mixture into the fillet with your hands, turning the fillet to pat the mixture onto both sides.

Drop the fillets into the very hot skillet and cook on each side for 3 to 4 minutes, being careful not to break the fillets when turning them over.

The tuna will look charred or "blackened." There may be some smoke, but it should not be excessive. The blackening forms a

(continued)

crunchy and spicy coating, sealing in the flavor as well as the moisture. Cook for at least 7 minutes, until the fish is no longer translucent and it is cooked all the way through.

Serve warm with lemon slices.

Southern Crusty
Herb Blend Coating

PREP TIME: 10 minutes
COOK TIME: none

PORTIONS: 5 (1 tablespoon each)
CARBS PER SERVING: ½ gram

Don't let the long list of herbs and spices discourage you. Include only as many as you have on hand, and chances are, you'll still love this crusty coating.

1 teaspoon ground ginger
1 teaspoon dried marjoram
1 teaspoon dried oregano
1 teaspoon dried rosemary
1 teaspoon dried sage
1 teaspoon dried thyme
1 teaspoon dried basil
3 teaspoons parsley flakes

1 teaspoon garlic powder
1 teaspoon onion flakes
1 teaspoon dried paprika (hot or sweet)
1 teaspoon cayenne (optional)
1 teaspoon salt
1 teaspoon pepper

Place all the ingredients in a blender. Blend on high speed until the spices become a fine powder. Store in an airtight container such as a screw-top jar.

Use the coating liberally as an all-purpose rub for grilled steaks, ribs, chops, poultry, and fish.

It's also excellent as a marinade when mixed with vinegar and oil (1 tablespoon herb blend, ½ cup white vinegar, 1 cup olive oil).

Crystal River Fried Steak

PREP TIME: 2 minutes	SERVINGS: 4
COOK TIME: 32 minutes	CARBS PER SERVING: 1 gram

One day while snorkeling in the Crystal River in central Florida, we were approached by a mother manatee and her calf. She stayed with us for almost an hour, circling and approaching, as curious about, and apparently appreciative of, us as we were interested in her and her baby. We thought we were too excited to eat that night, until we came across a little diner that served up a perfect Southern ending for a perfect Southern day. Here's our version.

1 tablespoon Southern Crusty Herb Blend Coating (page 119)
2 cups crushed pork rinds
2 eggs, beaten well

4 beef steaks (4 ounces each) or any well-marbled, boneless cut, 3/4 inch thick
4 tablespoons olive oil

Combine the Southern Crusty Herb Blend Coating and crushed pork rinds in a Ziploc plastic bag. Crush and mix. Remove to a plate.

Place the beaten eggs in a wide, shallow bowl.

Dip the steaks in the egg mixture to coat all sides, then dip them in the herb mixture. Press the coating into both sides of each steak with your hands.

In a large skillet, heat 2 tablespoons of the olive oil over a medium flame. When the oil is hot (not smoking), gently place 2 steaks into the oil and cook on one side, undisturbed, for about 7 minutes. Using a spatula, carefully turn the steaks, preserving the coating. Cook them on the other side for an additional 8 to 9 minutes, until cooked through.

Repeat this process with the remaining steaks and olive oil.

Serve the steaks warm with low-carb salad and vegetables.

EXOTIC
PLEASURES

Scottish Chicken in Mushroom Cream Sauce

PREP TIME: 20 minutes
COOK TIME: 65 minutes

SERVINGS: 4
CARBS PER SERVING: 3 grams

About eight miles north of Forfar, in Eastern Scotland, there's a little bed-and-breakfast that overlooks some of the greenest paddocks in the world. For a small "tariff," guests can purchase a three-course dinner that, alone, is well worth the trip. Our hosts Michael and Sonny used Rock Cornish hens in their version of this old family recipe, but we've found that chicken is just as good.

2 pounds chicken breast halves, boneless and skinless, cut into 1-inch cubes
4 tablespoons olive oil
6 medium mushrooms, sliced
4 cloves garlic, minced
1 cup cottage cheese

1 cup sour cream
2 tablespoons chopped fresh basil
1/2 tablespoon dried marjoram
1/2 teaspoon Dijon mustard
Salt and ground black pepper, as desired

Sauté the chicken cubes in the oil in a medium-size skillet over a medium-high flame. Stir and lift the chicken so that all the surfaces brown (about 10 minutes total). Remove the skillet from the heat and transfer the chicken to a 4-quart ovenproof casserole dish, leaving the drippings in the pan.

Preheat the oven to 350°F.

Transfer the mushroom slices and garlic to the skillet and heat them over a medium flame, stirring constantly until they are well cooked and turn a deep golden brown. Remove the skillet from the heat and allow the mushrooms and garlic to cool.

Place all the remaining ingredients in a blender and purée for 1 minute. Transfer the cottage cheese mixture to the skillet with the cooled mushrooms and drippings. Stir well.

Pour the mixture over the chicken pieces in the casserole dish,

(continued)

covering all exposed surfaces. Lift the pieces and turn them to ensure that all surfaces make contact with the creamy mixture.

Bake the chicken for 50 minutes or until cooked throughout.

Serve warm.

Piccadilly Circus Sirloin Steaks

PREP TIME: 5 minutes
COOK TIME: 20 minutes

SERVINGS: 4
CARBS PER SERVING: 2 grams

The sign in the café window in Piccadilly, London's famous shopping and entertainment center, announced "New-York-City-Style Burgers." They were served up on a plate instead of a bun, accompanied by spaghetti rather than fries, and green pepper slices in place of dill pickles. Although baffled by this interpretation of New York style, we were inspired to invent these chopped steaks, which surprised us with their richness and unusual blend of flavors.

1½ pounds ground sirloin
½ cup grated cheese (cheddar, American, Swiss, or Monterey Jack)
¼ cup crumbled blue cheese
2 slices bacon, cooked crisp and crumbled (optional)
1 teaspoon soy sauce

1 clove garlic, minced
1 teaspoon white vinegar or lemon juice
¼ cup chopped fresh parsley
Salt and pepper, as desired
2 teaspoons olive oil
½ green bell pepper, julienne
¼ cup chopped onion (optional)

Divide the beef into 8 parts and shape it into patties, each about 4 inches in diameter.

Combine the cheeses, bacon, soy sauce, garlic, vinegar or lemon juice, parsley, and salt and pepper in a small bowl; toss gently to blend well.

Mound one quarter of the cheese mixture onto each of the 4 patties. Top each mound with a second patty, pinching the edges together to seal.

Heat the oil in a medium-size nonstick skillet over a medium-high flame until hot (but not smoking).

Add the pepper strips and chopped onion; cook and stir the vegetables until the edges of the onion start to brown.

Remove the peppers and onion from the skillet to a plate. Cover them to keep them moderately warm.

Add the beef patties to the same skillet and cook over a medium-high flame for 8 minutes on the first side, until well browned.

(continued)

Turn the patties carefully and cook for at least 8 more minutes, until well done throughout (so that no pink remains inside).

Top the patties with the peppers and onion bits and serve immediately. These are great cold, too, especially wrapped in large, crisp lettuce leaves.

Belgian Sausage and Endive Soup

PREP TIME: 15 minutes
COOK TIME: 36 minutes

SERVINGS: 4 (1 cup each)
CARBS PER SERVING: 4 grams

The unusual blend of meat and sweet spices in this dish makes it a natural for holiday meals.

2 tablespoons unsalted butter
1/4 cup chopped onion
1 cup chopped celery
2 scallions, sliced thin
4 large endives, cored and chopped
12 patties sausage (or our Freedom Sausage, page 23), each patty quartered
4 cups chicken broth (or our Classic Chicken Stock, page 66)

1/2 teaspoon ground nutmeg
1/2 teaspoon ground cinnamon
Salt and pepper, as desired
1/2 cup heavy whipping cream
2 teaspoons arrowroot powder dissolved in 4 teaspoons of water (for thickening), optional
Parsley as garnish (optional)

Place a large soup pot over a medium flame. Melt the butter in the pot and sauté onion, celery, scallions, and chopped endive.

Stir the vegetables often until they become soft but not browned (4 minutes).

Add half of the sausage quarters and sauté for 2 more minutes.

Add the chicken broth and the remaining sausage quarters, and simmer, partially covered, for 30 minutes. Remove from the heat.

Season the mixture with nutmeg and cinnamon. Add salt and pepper, as desired.

Transfer batches of the soup mixture to a food processor or blender. Purée until smooth.

Add the cream and reheat the mixture over a medium flame until it's warm but not hot. Do not bring the mixture to a boil. Remove it from the heat and serve.

If a thicker soup is desired, add the arrowroot mixture after the soup has been removed from the heat. Stir constantly to make certain the arrowroot mixture is distributed throughout.

Garnish the soup with parsley, and serve.

Ginger Cream Shrimp

PREP TIME: 10 minutes	SERVINGS: 4
COOK TIME: 20 minutes	CARBS PER SERVING: 2 grams

Seven days on a scuba cruise, three dives a day, and you build up quite an appetite. Still, for us it was unthinkable to consider eating fish when we had been admiring them all day. John, the chef, was gracious enough to defrost some shrimp just for us (though we suspected they were meant as bait), and he whipped up a favorite he had been given by a local gourmet. Back home, we recreated his dish in our own way.

1 portobello mushroom,
  sliced
2 teaspoons olive oil
1 pound large shrimp,
  cleaned, shelled, and
  deveined
3 scallions, diced
2 tablespoons peeled and
  finely grated fresh ginger
  root

6 tablespoons heavy
  whipping cream
1 cup chicken stock (or our
  Classic Chicken Stock,
  page 66)
  Salt and pepper, as desired

Place a large skillet over a medium flame. Sauté the mushroom slices in the olive oil for 3 minutes, until softened.

Add the shrimp and heat, stirring often, until they are cooked through and no longer translucent—for at least 6 minutes. Remove the shrimp and cover to keep them moderately warm.

Place the scallions, ginger, and cream in the skillet. Heat slowly over a low flame, stirring constantly. As the cream mixture begins to warm, slowly add the chicken stock in a thin stream, stirring constantly. Heat the mixture well but not to the boiling point.

Add the shrimp and continue to cook, stirring, until the mixture is thick, about 3 minutes. Adjust seasoning with salt and pepper.

French Brussels Sprouts

PREP TIME: 8 minutes

COOK TIME: 13 minutes

SERVINGS: 4

CARBS PER SERVING: 3 grams

(with Madeira) 1 gram (without Madeira)

In the north of France, the locals serve a vegetable dish that makes American-style boiled vegetables pale in comparison. We thought it odd to see brussels sprouts on a French menu until we learned that the little green bundles of vitamin C were cultivated and developed primarily by the French and Belgians who provided them with their name.

1/4 pound (1 stick) butter

4 cloves fresh garlic, chopped fine

20 brussels sprouts, each split in half

1 tablespoon chopped fresh parsley

1 tablespoon chopped fresh basil

1 1/2 cups chicken stock (or our Classic Chicken Broth, page 66)

1/4 cup dessert wine such as Madeira (optional)

1/4 teaspoon salt

Place the butter in a small saucepan and melt it over low heat until it begins to brown.

Add the chopped garlic and sauté until the garlic is light brown.

Add the brussels sprouts and sauté for approximately 1 minute. Add the parsley, basil, chicken stock, dessert wine, and salt. Cook uncovered until the liquid is reduced somewhat and forms a buttery sauce (about 4 minutes). Remove from the heat and, using a slotted spoon, transfer the brussels sprouts to a serving dish.

Serve warm with as much of the sauce as you wish.

Kilkenny Chowder

PREP TIME: 8 minutes
COOK TIME: 90 minutes

SERVINGS: 4 (2½ cups each)
CARBS PER SERVING: 2 grams

Richard: *Our neighbor Sean Eagan, fresh from Kilkenny, Ireland, was new to Block Island, Rhode Island. When he heard that Rachael was fighting a powerful flu, Sean brought over a soup his mother and aunts always made when he was a child. If there's anything better than a good bowl of chowder when you're feeling low, it's one served up with a good helping of Irish generosity.*

1 pound white fish fillets (such as flounder, sole, etc.)
2 tablespoons olive oil
¼ cup chopped onion
2 cloves garlic, minced
¼ cup diced fresh tomato
1 cup sliced mushrooms
4 stalks celery, chopped
1 teaspoon salt
¼ teaspoon cayenne pepper (optional)
1 bay leaf

4 cups chicken stock (or our Classic Chicken Stock, page 66)
1 pound kale (or collards or turnip greens), washed, trimmed of coarse stems and veins, then thinly sliced
2 teaspoons arrowroot powder dissolved in 4 teaspoons of water, for thickening (optional)

Cut the fish fillets into 2-inch bite-size pieces.

In a large stockpot, heat the oil over a medium flame, tilting the pot to cover the bottom.

Fry the onion and garlic in the pot for 5 minutes. Add the tomato, mushrooms, celery, salt, cayenne, and bay leaf and cook, stirring constantly, for 5 minutes.

Add the chicken stock and bring to a boil. Reduce the heat and cover. Simmer for 1 hour.

Add the fish. Cook for 10 minutes.

Add the kale and simmer uncovered for 5 minutes, until the kale is tender and the color of jade.

When the fish is fully cooked and flakes easily with a fork, remove the pot from the heat.

Remove the bay leaf.

(continued)

If desired, add the arrowroot and water mixture for thickening. Stir constantly to make certain the arrowroot mixture is distributed throughout.

Serve the chowder warm.

Damyanti's Curried Salad

PREP TIME: 7 minutes
COOK TIME: none

SERVINGS: 4
CARBS PER SERVING: 2 grams

As professors at Mt. Sinai's Medical Center in New York, we mentored Damyanti, a young medical student from India. She never failed to bring a bowl of food to share at the Student Lunch Conference each Thursday. Other students, embarrassed at having brought sandwiches only for themselves, began to follow suit. In a matter of weeks, the meeting became a potluck celebration, a tradition that continues to this day. Here's our version of one of her salads.

Dressing

1 clove garlic
1/4 teaspoon peeled and thinly sliced fresh ginger root
2 tablespoons fresh lemon juice

1/2 teaspoon curry powder (or as desired)
1 teaspoon Dijon mustard
Salt and pepper, as desired
1/2 cup olive oil

Salad

3 to 4 cups leftover chicken, lamb, turkey, or other protein, cut into bite-size chunks
1 cup cauliflower florets, plunged into boiling water for 1 minute

1 cup sliced celery
4 cups spinach that has been washed well and torn into bite-size pieces

To make the dressing, place the garlic, ginger, lemon juice, curry, mustard, and salt and pepper as desired in a food processor and process well. Add the olive oil in a steady stream through the access tube while processing until smooth.

Refrigerate the dressing in a covered container for up to one day.

Place the salad ingredients in a large bowl and toss to mix well. Drizzle the dressing onto the salad and toss thoroughly to distribute evenly.

Chill, covered, for 1 hour before serving.

Chicken Salad Anise

PREP TIME: 10 minutes

COOK TIME: none

SERVINGS: 4

CARBS PER SERVING: 3 grams

Amid dozens of restaurants on Crete, we found a quiet and cool haven, a tiny place that served a small selection of authentic Greek dishes prepared by and for the island locals. We make it a practice to order two different meals so that we can share with each other, but when we saw this dish on the menu, we knew we each needed to order our own. Here's our interpretation of that authentic experience.

6 cups 3/4-inch cubes of cooked chicken
2 ounces feta cheese
4 tablespoons ricotta cheese
1/4 cup diced onion
1/4 cup pitted whole black ripe olives, drained and diced

1/2 tablespoon anise seeds
1/4 cup fresh mint leaves
6 romaine leaves
1 lemon, thinly sliced, as garnish (optional)

Place all the ingredients except the romaine leaves and lemon in a food processor. Process on a low setting for a few seconds until the mixture becomes a chunky blend.

Turn the mixture onto a bed of fresh romaine lettuce and serve surrounded by lemon slices as a garnish.

Mexican Swordfish

PREP TIME: 10 minutes
COOK TIME: 15 minutes

SERVINGS: 4
CARBS PER SERVING: 2 grams

In Venezuela, Pabellon con Baranda is virtually the national dish. Unfortunately, three of its ingredients are high-carb. Our hosts in Caracas, feeling bad that we could not indulge in their usual dinner of welcome, made a version of this meal instead. We praised them highly on their country's fine cuisine, only to be informed that they had come across the recipe on their recent trip to Puerto Vallarta, Mexico.

6 cups chicken stock (or our Classic Chicken Stock, page 66)
1½ tablespoons pickling spice
4 4-ounce swordfish fillets, ½ inch thick
¼ cup thinly sliced onion
3 cloves garlic, minced
¼ cup white vinegar

1 tablespoon olive oil
1¼ teaspoons dried cumin
1 tablespoon dried basil
1 tablespoon parsley flakes
1 green bell pepper, thinly sliced
2 tablespoons finely minced fresh red or green chili peppers

In a large saucepan over a medium-high flame bring the chicken stock and pickling spice to a boil. Continue a gentle rolling boil, partially covered, for 10 minutes.

Add the fish fillets, onion, garlic, vinegar, olive oil, cumin, basil, parsley, and green pepper. The fillets should be completely covered by the stock.

Simmer at a slow boil for about 5 minutes, until the fish is opaque and cooked throughout. Transfer the fish mixture to a serving plate. Drizzle the cooking liquid on the fish and top with minced chili peppers.

Tasmanian Calamari

PREP TIME: 10 minutes

COOK TIME: 6 minutes

SERVINGS: 4

CARBS PER SERVING: 1 gram

We took off for Hobart, Tasmania, without first checking on the weather. We left a sunny ninety-degree day to fly into a cold, rainy day, with a week of similar weather guaranteed. After we shivered through the prison tour at Port Arthur, there was virtually nothing else to do. The little restaurant across the street from our hotel surprised us with a warm welcome and the best food that two disappointed travelers could ask for. Over dinner, we decided to "cut bait and run," and return to Hobart a lot earlier in the summer of the following year, when the weather promised to be fine. Here's our version of that hotel welcome meal.

1 pound squid, cleaned, bodies and tentacles left whole

1 teaspoon soy sauce

1/4 cup finely chopped onion

1 teaspoon peeled and finely grated fresh ginger root

1/8 teaspoon cayenne (or as desired)

1 teaspoon Dijon mustard

2 teaspoons minced garlic

1/4 teaspoon salt

1/4 cup finely chopped fresh cilantro

Bring to a boil 2 quarts of water and 2 teaspoons of salt in a large saucepan over medium-high heat.

Drop the squid into the boiling water and stir constantly, until the squid is opaque and thoroughly cooked (approximately 2 minutes at a rolling boil).

Drain the squid in a colander and drench with cool running water to stop the cooking process. Cut the tentacles into bite-size pieces. Halve the bodies lengthwise, then cut them crosswise into thin strips.

Pour the remaining ingredients into very large mixing bowl and whisk well.

Add the drained squid and toss well to cover.

Serve immediately or after chilling.

Stuffed Kohlrabi

PREP TIME: 15 minutes
COOK TIME: 30 minutes

SERVINGS: 4
CARBS PER SERVING: 4 grams

Kohlrabi is often found in German recipes. It works so well in so many recipes, it's fast becoming an American favorite. Many supermarkets now stock kohlrabi in their produce departments, and if yours doesn't, it can probably be ordered for you. Try it. We can all use a new vegetable in our repertoire.

4 bulbs kohlrabi, peeled
1 tablespoon olive oil
1/4 cup chopped onion
1 cup crushed pork rinds
   Salt, pepper, and hot sauce,
   as desired

Parsley sprigs as garnish
(optional)
1 teaspoon arrowroot powder
   dissolved in 4 teaspoons of
   water, for thickening
   (optional)

Place the kohlrabi bulbs in a medium saucepan and cover with water. Cook over a high flame, covered, until they yield to a fork prick but are not mushy (about 15 minutes). Drain and cool. Set aside.

Trim 1/4 inch from the root end of the kohlrabies. Scoop out the pulp from the root end and set it aside. Scoop out the pulp from the opposite end and add it to the other pulp, leaving only the kohlrabi shells (about 1/4 inch thick).

Oil an ovenproof baking dish and set it aside.

Preheat the oven to 350°F.

In a medium-size bowl, mash the kohlrabi pulp, then add the onion and pork rinds. Toss to blend well.

Stuff the kohlrabi shells with the mixture and arrange the shells in the baking dish. Bake uncovered for 15 minutes, until the mixture begins to take on a texture similar to turkey stuffing.

Turn the oven off. Using a spatula to keep the mixture from leaking out of the bottom of the bulbs, transfer the kohlrabi to a serving plate. Retain the liquid from the bottom of the baking dish and add salt, pepper, and hot sauce as desired. If a thin sauce is preferred, drizzle the sauce on the stuffed kohlrabies, garnish with parsley, and serve immediately.

(continued)

If a thick sauce is desired, transfer the reserved and seasoned liquid to a small bowl and add the arrowroot mixture. Stir constantly to make certain the arrowroot mixture is distributed throughout. Drizzle the thickened sauce on the stuffed kohlrabies and serve immediately.

Seven-Mile Beach Jerk Pork

PREP TIME: 15 minutes
COOK TIME: 15 to 25 minutes

SERVINGS: 4
CARBS PER SERVING: 4 grams

Grand Cayman Island has some of the best scuba diving in the world. We love to visit just before the hurricane season, when the crowds have thinned out and the water is extra warm. Captain Hook's Restaurant at the Treasure Island Resort is actually several different restaurants under one roof. The various managements, working together, offer customers three menus to choose from. You can get your favorite Greek, American, and Island dishes served on one plate. We took our inspiration from this local favorite for the recipe below.

4 ½-inch-thick pork chops	2 teaspoons dried thyme
2 limes, juiced	1 teaspoon ground ginger
1 cup water	1 teaspoon salt
¼ cup minced onions	1½ teaspoons ground black
1½ cups minced scallions	pepper
6 cloves garlic, minced	3 tablespoons olive oil
2 teaspoons ground allspice	2 chopped fresh red or green
½ teaspoon ground nutmeg	chili peppers
1 tablespoon dried basil	

Place the pork in a large bowl. Cover with the lime juice and water. Refrigerate, covered, for 1 hour.

Transfer all the remaining ingredients to a blender or food processor and blend until the mixture becomes a smooth paste.

Add the paste to the bowl with the pork. Stir with your hands to make sure the paste mixes thoroughly with the lime juice and touches all surfaces of the pork. Cover and marinate the pork in the refrigerator for another 2 hours. Remove the pork from the refrigerator and discard all of the marinade.

Preheat an outdoor grill to medium-high heat. Lightly oil the grill grating.

Lay the pork chops across the preheated grill and cook, turning as needed to ensure even and thorough cooking.

Grill until the meat is well darkened on the outside and thoroughly cooked on the inside.

Portobellos Stuffed with Crab

PREP TIME: 8 minutes
COOK TIME: 15 minutes

SERVINGS: 4
CARBS PER SERVING: 1 gram

In Venice, Florida, we ventured into a restaurant with gondola murals on the walls that boasted that it offered the finest cuisine "on the canal." At first glance, we were not impressed. Still, friends said that the food was as authentic and excellent as anyone could hope for, so we gave it a try. Our friends were right on both counts. Here's our version of their signature appetizer, which proved to be such a happy surprise.

8 ounces crabmeat (canned or fresh), fully cooked
4 diced scallions
1/3 cup mayonnaise
1/3 cup grated Parmesan cheese
1 teaspoon dried basil
1/4 teaspoon dried thyme

1/4 teaspoon dried oregano
Ground black pepper, as desired
4 portobello mushrooms
1/4 teaspoon paprika (hot or sweet)
Lemon wedges, for garnish

Preheat the oven to 350°F.

In a medium-size bowl, combine the crabmeat, scallions, mayonnaise, 1/4 cup of the grated Parmesan, the basil, thyme, oregano, and pepper as desired. Hand mix to ensure complete blending.

Fill the inverted portobello caps with rounded spoonfuls of filling and place the mushrooms, filling side up, on a lightly greased baking sheet. Sprinkle the tops with the remaining Parmesan and the paprika.

Bake for 15 minutes.

Serve warm with lemon wedges.

Curried Okra with Gingered "Rice"

PREP TIME: 7 minutes
COOK TIME: 20 minutes

SERVINGS: 4
CARBS PER SERVING: 2 grams

Mention the word "okra" and people assume you're talking about Southern cooking. Actually, this unusual and low-carb vegetable comes from Northern Africa. Because it releases a sticky juice, okra thickens sauces and stews and virtually any dish in which it is included. This Indian-style curry will surprise you with its aromatic blend of flavors, while it fortifies you with a good helping of vitamins A and C and folate. When you need a low-carb "thickener" for your next low-carb dish, think okra.

7 tablespoons olive oil	1/4 cup chopped onion
1/2 teaspoon peeled and finely grated fresh ginger root	1/2 teaspoon cayenne (or hot sauce)
1/2 head small cauliflower, grated roughly (approximately 2 1/2 cups)	1/4 teaspoon ground turmeric
	1/4 teaspoon curry powder
	Salt and pepper, as desired
1 pound fresh okra	1/2 cup mint leaves, as garnish (optional)

Heat 4 tablespoons of the olive oil in a large skillet or wok over medium heat.

Add the ginger root and stir-fry for 1 minute.

Add the cauliflower and stir-fry for 6 minutes, mixing constantly. Remove from the heat and transfer to a serving plate. Allow the cauliflower to cool uncovered.

Wash the okra, trim the ends, and slice it into half-inch pieces. Dry with paper towels.

Heat the remaining 3 tablespoons of olive oil in a medium-size skillet over a medium flame until hot (but not smoking). Add the okra and sauté for 7 minutes, stirring often to prevent sticking.

Add the onion and continue to sauté for 3 more minutes.

When the okra begins to brown, add the cayenne, turmeric, curry

(continued)

powder, and salt and pepper as desired. Continue to sauté and stir for an additional 2 minutes.

Pour the okra mixture over the cauliflower and garnish with the mint. (Do not rewarm the cauliflower "rice." It will stay crunchy if it remains at room temperature.)

Beausoleil Bouillabaisse

PREP TIME: 15 minutes
COOK TIME: 1 hour, 10 minutes

SERVINGS: 5 (1 cup each)
CARBS PER SERVING: 3 grams per cup

Neither of us ever thought the idea of "fish soup" sounded appealing until we tasted it in a little bistro in the southern French town of Beausoleil, sipping it slowly as we basked in the evening breeze, the coast of Monaco visible in the distance. Now this version of the dish has become a classic in our home, served up in big cups with a bit of Gruyère cheese melted on top.

2 cloves garlic, crushed
2 tablespoons olive oil
1 small onion, chopped
3 scallions, chopped
1/2 small tomato, chopped
1 1/2 pounds fish in any combination (swordfish, halibut, flounder, sea bass, etc.), carefully deboned, cut into 2-inch chunks
4 cups fish stock (or our Fundamental Fish Stock, page 185)

2 bay leaves
1/4 cup chopped fresh parsley
1/2 teaspoon dried rosemary
1 teaspoon dried basil
Salt and black pepper, as desired
2 teaspoons arrowroot powder dissolved in 4 teaspoons of water, for thickening (optional)
3 ounces Gruyère cheese, sliced thin (optional)

Sauté the garlic in the olive oil in a large soup pot over a medium flame. Stir constantly.

Add the onions, scallions, and tomato and sauté for 4 minutes, until they begin to soften.

Add half of the fish and heat, stirring constantly, turning so that all surfaces of the fish make contact with the heated oil and vegetable mixture.

Add the fish stock, bay leaves, parsley, rosemary, basil, and salt and pepper as desired. Stir well and bring to a boil.

Partially cover and cook at a slow rolling boil until the broth has reduced and thickened (approximately 30 minutes).

Add the remaining fish. Continue to cook in the same way for 30 minutes more.

(continued)

Remove from the heat and carefully take out the bay leaves.

If desired, add the arrowroot and water mixture for thickening. Stir constantly to make certain the arrowroot mixture is distributed throughout.

Serve the bouillabaisse warm. If you would like a chewy cheese topping on it, pour individual servings into ovenproof bowls and top with a slice or two of Gruyère cheese. Place the servings under the broiler for 1 minute, until the cheese melts and turns golden brown.

HEARTY
FEASTS

Chicken with Green Cheese

PREP TIME: 10 minutes
COOK TIME: 1 hour

SERVINGS: 4
CARBS PER SERVING: 2 grams

Originally a Greek mainstay, this main course lends itself to new variations every time we make it. This is our latest version, but chances are, even as you're making it you'll find extra ingredients you want to add, too.

1/4 teaspoon salt	3 tablespoons olive oil
1/4 teaspoon pepper	2 cloves garlic, minced
1 tablespoon fresh basil	2 green bell peppers, cored,
1/2 teaspoon dried sage	seeded, sliced thin
1 teaspoon dried rosemary	2 tablespoons soy sauce
6 ounces feta cheese,	Wooden toothpicks
crumbled (or ricotta	Lemon wedges or parsley,
cheese)	for garnish (optional)
4 chicken breast halves,	
boneless and skinless,	
pounded thin for rolling	

In a medium-size bowl, mix the salt, pepper, basil, sage, and rosemary. Add the feta cheese a few tablespoons at a time, mixing thoroughly.

Divide the cheese mixture into 4 portions and spread it evenly on top of each piece of chicken. Place the chicken in the refrigerator while you prepare the green peppers.

Preheat the oven to 350°F.

In a small skillet, warm the olive oil over a medium flame until hot (but not smoking). Add the garlic and stir constantly for 1 minute. Add the green pepper slices and cook for 6 minutes, until soft, stirring often.

Remove the chicken breasts from the refrigerator. Place the green pepper slices evenly across the breasts and sprinkle with soy sauce.

Roll the chicken breasts into logs, secure with toothpicks, and place them seam side down on an oiled baking sheet.

Bake for 50 minutes, until the chicken is cooked throughout and the meat is no longer pink at all.

Remove the toothpicks and serve warm, garnished with lemon wedges or fresh parsley as desired.

Almost Potatoes Au Gratin

PREP TIME: 13 minutes
COOK TIME: 32 minutes

SERVINGS: 4
CARBS PER SERVING: 4 grams

This dish is great as part of a Sunday brunch or all alone as a filling snack.

1 head cauliflower, florets only
2 tablespoons butter
4 ounces cream cheese
2 scallions, diced
Salt and black pepper, as desired

Cayenne pepper or hot sauce, as desired
6 slices bacon, cooked crisp, then diced
4 ounces cheese (American and cheddar melt best), grated

Preheat the oven to 350°F.

In a deep skillet over a high flame, bring 1½ inches of water to a boil. Add the cauliflower and boil for exactly 3 minutes. Turn off the heat, pour off the water, and cover. Put aside.

Blend the butter, cream cheese, scallions, and salt and pepper and hot sauce or cayenne as desired in a large mixing bowl.

Add the cauliflower to the cream cheese mixture a cup at a time. Toss to coat the cauliflower.

Transfer the coated cauliflower to a shallow ovenproof casserole dish. Sprinkle the bacon evenly over the cauliflower and top with one layer of cheese.

Bake for 20 to 25 minutes, until the cheese is melted.

Edmonton Pork and Beans

PREP TIME: 7 minutes

COOK TIME: 28 minutes

SERVINGS: 4

CARBS PER SERVING: 4 grams

The storm hit Snow Valley with an intensity that no one expected. We thought we could make the last bus out, but it was canceled just as we were paying for our tickets. We were grateful to get the last room at a nearby hotel and even more appreciative when our hosts made a hearty meal for all the stranded travelers. It was not what we anticipated when we were told they were serving "pork and beans," but we've been making our version of it ever since.

1½ pounds green beans (or wax or snap beans), trimmed

3 tablespoons olive oil

2 cloves garlic, minced

4 thin pork chops (no more than ½ inch thick)

8 tablespoons sour cream

1 tablespoon Dijon mustard

½ teaspoon salt

Hot sauce, as desired

1 cup grated sharp cheddar cheese

Preheat the oven to 350°F.

Fill a deep skillet with 1½ inches of water. Bring the water to a boil over a high flame. Add the green beans and boil for 3 minutes exactly.

Remove from the heat, drain, and cover. Put aside.

Warm the olive oil in a large skillet over a medium-high flame until hot (but not smoking). Add garlic and pork chops and cook until the chops are browned (about 4 minutes), then turn and brown the other side (an additional 4 minutes).

Remove from the heat, retaining drippings in the skillet, and transfer the chops to a shallow ovenproof casserole dish, large enough to accommodate all of them in a single layer. (The chops must be placed in a single layer to ensure thorough cooking).

Place an equal proportion of green beans over each chop. Put aside.

Add the sour cream, mustard, salt, and hot sauce as desired to the cooled skillet drippings and mix and scrape to blend flavors.

Pour the sauce over the green beans and chops.

Top with the grated cheese.

Place in the oven and bake uncovered for 20 minutes, until the pork is cooked throughout.

Serve warm.

Herb-Encrusted Steak

PREP TIME: 3 minutes
COOK TIME: 19 minutes

SERVINGS: 4
CARBS PER SERVING: 1 gram

The two secrets to getting a great crust are (1) lay on the ingredients in exactly the order recommended and (2) do not disturb the coating once it has been laid down. We love these fillets cold as a great late-night snack with celery sticks.

2 steaks, rib eye, strip, or any
   well-marbled cut, boneless,
   about 10 ounces each, cut
   down the middle to form
   2 fillets each
3 tablespoons Dijon mustard

1/2 teaspoon dried thyme
1/4 teaspoon ground ginger
1 teaspoon dried basil
2 teaspoons garlic powder
1 tablespoon paprika (sweet
   or hot)

Preheat the broiler.

Place the steaks on a broiler pan and broil for 8 minutes.

Remove the pan from the oven and turn the steaks over.

Carefully brush mustard on the upper (raw) side of steak, covering all exposed surfaces.

One by one, sprinkle each of the herbs onto the mustard-covered surfaces.

Place the pan under the broiler with the steaks mustard side up and broil for 8 minutes more. Watch carefully to avoid burning.

Serve warm or cold.

Independence Day Flounder

PREP TIME: 6 minutes
COOK TIME: 20 minutes

SERVINGS: 4
CARBS PER SERVING: 4 grams

It had been a particularly hectic week. No time to shop for food and barely enough time to eat it. By the time the weekend came, we had used up almost all of our pre-made freezer meals, and assumed we'd stock up the kitchen on Saturday. But it was July 4 and our supermarket (and almost every other food store in the area) had closed at noon. When we faced the empty store at two in the afternoon, we realized we'd better be inventive with whatever food we had in the house. Here's the dish we threw together and have been enjoying ever since.

4   tablespoons olive oil
1/2 cup chopped scallions
4   fresh or defrosted flounder
    fillets (4 to 6 ounces each)
    about 1 inch thick, carefully
    deboned
2   stalks celery, diced
2   teaspoons lemon zest

1/2 teaspoon dried tarragon
12 pitted whole green olives,
    drained and diced
1/3 cup chicken stock (or our
    Classic Chicken Stock,
    page 66)
    Salt and pepper, as desired
3/4 cup sour cream

In a large skillet over a medium flame, heat 3 tablespoons of the olive oil until hot (but not smoking).

Preheat the oven to 200°F.

Add the scallions to the skillet and sauté until tender (about 3 minutes).

Add the fish fillets and cook on one side until brown and well cooked (about 4 minutes). Turn each fillet gently and continue to cook until the fish is cooked and opaque throughout (4 to 6 more minutes). Remove the skillet from the heat and transfer the fillets to an ovenproof plate. Cover and place in the oven to keep warm.

Return the skillet to medium heat, adding one tablespoon of the olive oil, the celery, and the lemon zest. Stir well, mixing with the drippings from the fish. Heat for 1 to 2 minutes, until the celery softens, stirring constantly.

Add the dried tarragon and green olives. Stir well.

(continued)

Slowly add the chicken stock, stirring constantly and heating thoroughly (about 3 minutes). Add salt and pepper as desired.

Remove from heat and allow to cool for 3 minutes, still stirring constantly.

Add the sour cream, a dollop at a time, mixing after each addition.

Remove the fish from the oven and pour the sour cream mixture over the fillets.

Serve immediately.

Crock-Pot Tender Roast Beef

PREP TIME: 5 minutes

COOK TIME: 7 to 8 hours (Crock-Pot)

SERVINGS: 4

CARBS PER SERVING: 3 grams

We put this roast on to cook mid-morning, set the timer, and never think about it for hours. After you add the chicken stock (yes, it matches the beef flavor perfectly!), the only thing that demands your attention is the heavenly smell that keeps calling you to come eat.

1¼ pound boneless beef roast
    for pot roast
3 cloves garlic, thinly sliced
    Salt and pepper, as desired

2 cups chicken stock (or our
    Classic Chicken Stock,
    page 66)
2 tablespoons white prepared
    horseradish
2 tablespoons dried basil

Place the pot roast, fat side down, in a Crock-Pot.

Place the garlic slivers over the top of the roast and sprinkle lightly with salt and pepper as desired.

Set the Crock-Pot dial on low and let cook, covered, for 5 hours.

Combine the chicken stock and horseradish in a small saucepan over low heat. Add the basil, a bit at a time, mixing and heating constantly. Heat until hot (but not boiling).

Gently pour the chicken stock along the side of the Crock-Pot, allowing it to pool at the bottom. Lift the roast to ensure that the bottom of it makes contact with the stock.

Turn the dial to medium and cook an additional 2 to 3 hours. Check to see if the meat easily pulls apart and is cooked throughout.

Serve the meat with au jus gravy.

Tasty Turkey Burgers

PREP TIME: 5 minutes
COOK TIME: 15 minutes

SERVINGS: 4 (1 burger each)
CARBS PER SERVING: 1 gram

The grated cheese, herbs, and garlic in this recipe give these burgers a rich and delicious flavor. Add a dill pickle and you're all set!

1 pound ground turkey	2 tablespoons dried rosemary
2 eggs, beaten	2 tablespoons dried thyme
2 tablespoons soy sauce	1 teaspoon garlic powder (or
4 tablespoons grated Parmesan or Romano cheese	2 cloves garlic, crushed) Salt, pepper, and hot sauce, as desired
1/2 tablespoon dried sage	4 tablespoons olive oil
2 tablespoons dried basil	

In a large mixing bowl, combine the turkey, eggs, soy sauce, grated cheese, sage, basil, rosemary, thyme, garlic powder, salt, pepper, and hot sauce as desired. Mix well with your hands to ensure an even distribution of all ingredients.

Form into four patties, about 3 inches across and 3/4 inch thick.

Refrigerate covered for at least 2 hours to allow flavors to blend.

Heat the olive oil in a large skillet, over a medium flame, until the oil is hot (but not smoking).

Carefully add the patties (they may spurt hot oil) to the oil and cook until brown and well done on one side (about 7 minutes).

Turn and cook on the other side until well browned and thoroughly cooked (7 to 8 minutes).

Serve hot or cold.

Canadian Logger Stew

PREP TIME: 7 minutes
COOK TIME: 2 hours

SERVINGS: 4
CARBS PER SERVING: 2 grams

We first had this deeply satisfying stew in a real-life logging camp. We got lost on the highway in Manitoba, Canada (Rachael was navigating!). Although the owner of the only boardinghouse in the camp charged as much for our room as the best hotel in New York, we had no choice but to accept. For an additional small fortune, she threw in dinner and breakfast. Dinner was this stew, piping hot. It was delicious. Breakfast, we were speechless to find out, was the same stew served cold. Still, we ate it—and found it to be quite good! So good, in fact, that we came up with our own version—for dinner or breakfast.

2 tablespoons butter
1 tablespoon olive oil
1/4 cup finely chopped onion
1 1/4 pounds beef, boneless and cubed
5 mushrooms, sliced
1 tomato, peeled, seeded, and diced
1/4 cup dry white wine (optional)
1/2 teaspoon dried tarragon
1 tablespoon dried basil
1 tablespoon paprika (hot or sweet)

4 cups beef stock (or the Classic Beef Stock, a variation of our Classic Chicken Stock, page 66)
Salt and pepper, as desired
2 cups green beans (or wax or snap beans), trimmed
1 cup sliced green bell pepper (optional)
1 cup small mushroom caps
2 teaspoons arrowroot powder dissolved in 4 teaspoons of water, for thickening (optional)

Heat the butter and oil in a large skillet or stockpot, over a medium flame. Add the onion and cook, stirring constantly, for 3 minutes, until the onion edges turn brown.

Add the beef cubes and brown lightly on all sides (about 6 minutes). Add the sliced mushrooms and cook for 3 more minutes.

Add the tomato, wine, tarragon, basil, paprika, beef stock, and salt and pepper as desired. Bring to a boil, cover, reduce heat, and simmer until the beef is very tender (about 1 1/2 hours).

(continued)

Add the green beans, green pepper, and mushroom caps and cook, uncovered, 6 to 8 minutes, until the beans and green pepper are almost tender but still crisp.

Remove from heat. If desired, add the arrowroot and water mixture for thickening. Stir constantly to make certain the arrowroot mixture is distributed throughout.

Serve warm.

Chili Beef and Cheese

PREP TIME: 13 minutes
COOK TIME: 23 minutes

SERVINGS: 4
CARBS PER SERVING: 4 grams

Here's proof that even on a low-carb diet you can have a great bowl of chili. If we don't make double the recipe, we always regret it.

4 tablespoons olive oil
1/2 green bell pepper, diced
1 cup chopped celery
1/4 cup diced onion
1 scallion, finely diced
1 clove garlic, minced

1/4 small fresh red or green chili pepper*, diced, or hot sauce, as desired
1 pound ground beef
1/2 cup grated cheese (cheddar or American melt best)
Salt and pepper, as desired

Heat 2 tablespoons of the olive oil in a large skillet on a medium flame, making certain to cover the bottom of the skillet. Stirring often, sauté the green pepper, celery, onion, scallion, and garlic until the onion turns transparent and the green pepper and celery soften a bit (about 4 minutes).

Add the chili pepper. Sauté and stir for 1 minute, so that spicy flavor is distributed throughout.

Remove from heat, set aside, and allow to cool.

Place the ground beef a little at a time in a large mixing bowl, breaking up clumps of meat as you add it. Add the vegetable mixture, including drippings, and mix well, using your hands to ensure that all the ingredients are evenly distributed and well combined.

Transfer the meat mixture to a large skillet and cook over a medium-high flame, stirring constantly, until the meat is completely cooked (about 18 minutes).

Sprinkle the cheese evenly over the meat and stir.

Add salt and pepper as desired, and serve warm as a main dish

*NOTE: When handling chili peppers, it's always a good idea to wear rubber or latex gloves. The pepper can burn and irritate your hands even if you are not aware of any tiny cuts or abrasions that may exist. Be certain not to touch your face or eyes or any other area that may be vulnerable to damage or irritation. Immediately wash the knife, cutting surfaces, and gloves when finished.

(continued)

or spoon into lettuce or spinach leaves to create grab-and-go meat pockets.

VARIATION

For another great-tasting option: add layers of shredded lettuce and a dollop of sour cream to the meat mixture and serve as a filling for our Truly Low-Carb Wraps (page 94).

Sunday Dinner Roast Chicken

PREP TIME: 9 minutes

COOK TIME: 1 hour

SERVINGS: 6

CARBS PER SERVING: 2

When you walk into the Prime Time Café at Disney World in Orlando, you would swear you're back in the 1950s. The ambience, the menu, even the taste of the food is authentic. We always order their roast chicken. It reminds us of the Sunday dinners of another generation, when food was filling and comforting, and families always ate together. Here's our version of the dish that's as good as "the good old days."

1 (2 to 2½ pounds) chicken	1 green bell pepper, quartered
4 tablespoons olive oil	¼ cup thinly sliced onions
4 tablespoons dried rosemary	6 mushroom caps
4 tablespoons dried basil	2 scallions, split in half
1 teaspoon salt	4 stalks celery, split in half
1 teaspoon pepper	

Preheat the oven to 350°F.

Place the rack in a roasting pan filled with 1½ inches of water (so that the water does not touch the bottom of the rack).

Rinse the chicken inside and out under running water and pat dry with paper towels, then place it on a large plate and pour olive oil on the skin and all exposed surfaces.

Place the rosemary, basil, salt, and pepper into a medium-size shallow bowl and mix, then sprinkle the herb mixture evenly over all the oiled surfaces of the chicken to make a crust.

Place the chicken on the rack in the roasting pan and bake, uncovered, maintaining the 1½-inch water level in the roasting pan to catch drippings, for 30 minutes.

Place the remaining ingredients in the water at the bottom of roasting pan.

Bake, uncovered, for an additional 15 minutes, maintaining the 1½-inch water level in the roasting pan. Then bake, uncovered, for a final 15 minutes (1 hour total), allowing the water level to decrease to about half the original level in order to form a thicker, more flavorful au jus gravy.

(continued)

Remove the chicken from the oven and allow it to "breathe" for 10 minutes before carving.

Serve the chicken warm with roasted vegetables in au jus gravy.

Grits, Sausage, and Gravy

PREP TIME: 15 minutes
COOK TIME: 8 minutes

SERVINGS: 4
CARBS PER SERVING: 4 grams

Rachael: *I'd lived in apartments in New York City for most of my life when Richard and I moved into our first home. Having read our books, our neighbor, Sonny, welcomed us with a true Southern dish, made low-carb just for us. Here's our version of that delicious welcome dish.*

1 head cauliflower, florets only
1 teaspoon olive oil

1½ pounds sausage patties, fully cooked (or our Freedom Sausage, Old-Fashioned Variation, page 23, fully cooked)
1 cup sour cream

Preheat the oven to 250°F.

In a large saucepan over high heat, boil the cauliflower florets in 1½ inches of water for 4 minutes exactly.

Remove from heat, drain in a colander, and submerge the florets in cold water to stop cooking immediately. When the florets are cool enough to handle easily, transfer them to a cutting board.

Using a nonserrated knife, cut the florets until they take on a "riced" texture (tiny, non-mushy bits). Using a spatula, carefully scrape the riced cauliflower into a medium-size ovenproof casserole dish. Transfer the casserole, covered, to the oven.

In a medium-size skillet over a medium flame, heat the olive oil until just warm, not hot. Add the sausage, breaking each patty into eighths and stirring them into the warm olive oil. Reduce heat to low.

Slowly add dollops of the sour cream, one at a time, to the warm sausage mixture. Stir gently after each addition of sour cream.

When all the sour cream has been incorporated, warmed slightly, and mixed, remove the mixture from the heat and set aside.

Remove the casserole dish containing the riced cauliflower from the oven.

Pour the sausage mixture over the riced cauliflower. Toss gently to distribute the sausage and sour cream "gravy" throughout, and serve.

Roasted Green Pepper Sauce

PREP TIME: 20 minutes
COOK TIME: 4 minutes

SERVINGS: 4 (½ cup each)
CARBS PER SERVING: 3 grams

We love to serve this appetizer to our guests. Those on low-carb diets are thrilled to get a dish so delicious yet low-carb. Guests who are not on diets never suspect that this treat is low in carbs. You get to enjoy it anytime you want!

4 tablespoons olive oil
3 green bell peppers, cored, seeded, cut in ½-inch-wide strips
8 scallions, diced
¼ cup fresh cilantro leaves
2 cloves garlic, minced

8 ounces cream cheese, quartered and softened
¼ teaspoon salt
¼ teaspoon crushed red pepper or hot sauce, as desired

Preheat the broiler.

Pour the olive oil in a shallow bowl.

Dip each strip of green pepper into the olive oil and place it on a baking sheet.

Broil the pepper strips under the broiler for 4 minutes, or until the skins begin to brown all over (but are not burned).

Immediately remove from the oven and place the pepper strips in a paper bag. Seal the bag and allow the peppers to steam for 15 minutes. Open the paper bag and allow the pepper strips to cool.

When the peppers are cool enough to handle, peel away the skin and discard it. Set the peppers aside.

Place the scallions, cilantro, and garlic in a food processor or blender and process until finely chopped.

Add the roasted green peppers, process, then add the cream cheese, salt, and crushed pepper or hot sauce as desired. Process once again.

Serve immediately or refrigerate overnight. Use as a dip for meat, poultry, tofu, or vegetables, or as a flavor-filled snack with Crisp and Crackly Cheese Crackers (page 104).

Salmon Scones

PREP TIME: 6 minutes   SERVINGS: 4
COOK TIME: 25 minutes   CARBS PER SERVING: 2 grams

Breakfast in other countries includes a wide variety of breakfast food that most Americans would never consider eating first thing in the morning: spaghetti and broiled tomatoes in Australia and lamb in New Zealand, for example. In Nova Scotia, our hosts adapted their high-carb salmon scones to fit our low-carb needs. They were great— both the hosts and the scones!

Nonstick cooking spray
1 can (7.5 ounces) salmon, drained and flaked
2 eggs, well beaten
1/2 cup finely chopped green bell pepper
3 scallions, finely chopped
1/2 cup finely grated sharp cheddar

Preheat the oven to 350°F. Evenly coat a nonstick muffin pan with nonstick cooking spray.

Combine the remaining ingredients in a medium-size bowl, mixing well to blend the textures and flavors.

Place one quarter of the mixture in each of 4 muffin cups.

Bake until the mixture has set (about 25 minutes) and the egg is completely cooked.

Remove the scones from the oven and allow them to cool before using a butter knife to loosen them from the muffin cups.

Serve as a stick-to-the-ribs breakfast, as a snack, or as an appetizer.

ITALIAN INDULGENCES

Chicken Pavarotti

PREP TIME: 15 minutes

COOK TIME: 80 minutes

SERVINGS: 4

CARBS PER SERVING: 3 grams

Alice Tully Hall in New York City had just been refurbished. When the great tenor Luciano Pavarotti sang that Christmas Eve, his voice washed over us like a band of angels. At the gala following the performance, a superb dish, one of the tenor's favorites, was served. Each time we make our low-carb version, we are reminded of a performance that filled our hearts and our souls.

1/4 cup olive oil

4 (4 ounces each) chicken breast halves, boneless and skinless

1 onion, finely chopped

1 green bell pepper, cut into 1/2-inch strips

1 cup chopped celery

3 cloves garlic, finely minced

12 mushrooms, sliced

1/2 tomato, finely diced

1/4 cup dry red wine (optional)

2 bay leaves

1 teaspoon dried basil

2 cups water

Salt and pepper, as desired

Preheat the oven to 350°F.

Heat the olive oil in a large skillet over a medium-high flame until hot (not smoking).

Add the chicken breasts and brown on both sides (about 5 minutes on each side).

Remove the chicken from the pan, leaving drippings, and place in a large ovenproof casserole. Set aside.

Add the onion, green pepper, celery, garlic, mushrooms, and tomatoes to the skillet. Stir constantly and cook until the onion begins to brown around the edges.

Add the wine, bay leaves, and basil. Mix well and warm.

Slowly add the water, stirring constantly. Warm to blend flavors (not to the boiling point).

Pour the mixture over the chicken. Cover and bake for 30 minutes.

Uncover and bake for an additional 40 minutes, so that the chicken is done throughout (not pink at all) and the sauce thickens.

Remove the bay leaves.

Serve warm.

Pizza Crisps

PREP TIME: 5 minutes

COOK TIME: 2 minutes

SERVINGS: 4

CARBS PER SERVING: 5 grams

We were desperate for pizza and made up these snacks on the spot. Now we keep the ingredients in our refrigerator at all times . . . just in case.

2 green bell peppers, ice cold, cored, seeded, and cut in half lengthwise

8 sausage patties, fully cooked and halved (or our Freedom Sausage, page 23, fully cooked and halved)

1/2 tomato, finely diced

Oregano and garlic powder, as desired

1/2 cup grated mozzarella cheese

Grated Parmesan or Romano cheese, as desired (optional)

Preheat the broiler.

Arrange the four inverted green pepper halves on a baking tray.

Pile on, in order, the sausage patties, tomato bits, oregano and garlic powder as desired, and mozzarella, evenly dividing the ingredients among all 4 green pepper halves.

Place the peppers under the broiler for 2 minutes—long enough to melt the mozzarella but not to soften the green pepper.

Sprinkle with Parmesan or Romano cheese as desired, and serve immediately, while the mozzarella is still warm and dripping.

Napoli Meat Pies

PREP TIME: 5 minutes
COOK TIME: 10 minutes

SERVINGS: 4 (½ sandwiches)
CARBS PER SERVING: 2 grams

Rachael: *When I was five years old, I was taken under the wing of a young neighbor. Apparently, Angie wanted to adopt me (really adopt me), and since my parents seemed intent on keeping me as part of our family, she did the next best thing: she fed me and spoiled me every chance she got. Soon, imitating Angie, I would only eat and, as much as I could, speak Italian. This was one of my favorite snacks. Squisito!*

4　portobello mushrooms
2　tablespoons olive oil
2　cloves garlic, crushed
1　teaspoon dried oregano
1　teaspoon dried basil

¹/₄　pound ground beef
　　Salt and pepper, as desired
4　ounces mozzarella cheese,
　　cut into 4 slices

On a plate, invert 2 of the portobello mushrooms. Set aside.

Warm the olive oil in a medium-size skillet on a medium flame. Add the garlic, oregano, and basil. Stir and warm for about 2 minutes.

Add the ground beef and brown well, stirring constantly (about 6 minutes) so that all the meat is well cooked.

Add the salt and pepper as desired and mix well. Remove from heat.

Place a rounded tablespoon of browned meat into each of the 2 mushrooms and smooth out evenly.

Add 1 slice of cheese per mushroom, then one additional tablespoon of browned meat, to form layers.

Top each mushroom with another mushroom, smooth side up, to form a sandwich.

Return the mushroom "sandwiches" to the skillet and cook over a low flame to warm. Cover for 2 to 3 minutes to melt the cheese and soften the mushrooms. Turn the mushrooms over and cook, covered, for an additional 2 to 3 minutes.

Transfer the "sandwiches" back to the plate. Cut each in half or quarters.

Serve warm.

Tuna Chia Pets

PREP TIME: 5 minutes
COOK TIME: none

SERVINGS: 4
CARBS PER SERVING: 2 grams

We first came up with this dish as our contribution to a friends' pool party. This fun snack, our version of the traditional Italian treat, Polpette di Tonno, was meant for the adults' table, but when our friends' seven-year-old granddaughter wanted to taste it, we were happy to oblige. "They're good!" she announced, reaching for another. "Sort of like fishy Chia Pets."

2 cans (6½ ounces each) tuna in water, drained and flaked
¼ cup diced onion
¼ diced green bell pepper
6 pitted green olives, drained and sliced
6 pitted black ripe olives, drained and sliced

1 cup mayonnaise
1 teaspoon dried oregano
1 teaspoon dried basil
2 cups alfalfa sprouts
6 romaine lettuce leaves, washed, dried, and cut in half

Combine the tuna, onion, pepper, sliced olives, mayonnaise, oregano, and basil in a large bowl. Mix well with your hands to blend completely. The mixture should have the consistency of very moist tuna salad.

For ease of handling, place the mixture covered in the refrigerator for 1 hour.

Spread 1 cup of the alfalfa sprouts evenly on a plate. Arrange the lettuce leaf halves on another serving platter.

Remove the tuna mixture from the refrigerator. Divide the mixture into quarters, then divide each quarter into three equal parts.

Wet your hands and roll one of the twelve equal parts into a ball. Roll the ball in the sprouts, coating it completely. Place each tuna ball on one lettuce leaf half and then repeat the process, adding the rest of the alfalfa spouts to the plate as they are needed to coat the tuna balls.

Serve immediately. The lettuce leaf should act as a "wrap" around the tuna ball when cupped in a hand, for easy snacking.

(continued)

VARIATION

For a sharper, spicier taste, substitute large arugula leaves for the lettuce leaves.

Bronx Salami

PREP TIME: 13 minutes

COOK TIME: 1 hour

SERVINGS: 6 (6 slices each)

CARBS PER SERVINGS: 0 grams

We can't remember their names or even their faces, but we'll never forget their hospitality: A picnic in Van Cortlandt Park in the Bronx, given by friends of friends of friends, who wanted to say thank you for their success on our program. Everything on the menu was low-carb, a totally "legal" potluck meal with a whole host of new recipes for everyone to swap and enjoy.

2　pounds pork, beef, or turkey, boneless, ground well, with natural fat

3　cloves garlic (regular or elephant), minced

1　teaspoon black pepper

1/2　teaspoon mustard seeds

1　teaspoon paprika (hot or sweet)

1　teaspoon salt

1　teaspoon oregano (more if desired)

1　teaspoon dried basil

1　teaspoon parsley flakes

　　Hot sauce or crushed red pepper flakes, as desired

In a large bowl, mix all the ingredients well and shape into 2 or 3 logs, each the size and shape of a small salami. Wrap in aluminum foil and twist the ends very well.

With the foil covering still in place, slide the rolls into a large soup pot filled with boiling water. Cook at a slow rolling boil, uncovered, for 1 hour.

Remove the rolls from the water and punch holes in the foil to allow grease to drain. Rewrap the rolls in a second layer of foil and return them to the refrigerator for 2 hours.

Remove the foil. Slice the rolls into disks 1/4 inch thick and serve cold.

Enjoy as part of a chef's salad (with cheese, hard-boiled egg slices, and greens) or as a stuffing with romaine lettuce and mustard in one of our Truly Low-Carb Wraps (page 94). Also excellent in our Anytime Antipasto (page 175).

Chicken Parmesan Romana

PREP TIME: 8 minutes
COOK TIME: 12 minutes

SERVINGS: 4
CARBS PER SERVING: 3 grams

The idea of cabbage pasta may seem odd at first, but when you taste it and realize that we really taste what's on pasta a great deal more than what's in pasta, it will make a lot of sense to drop the carbs and keep the taste.

1/2 head cabbage, sliced into 1/2-inch-thick strips (about 5 cups raw)
2 tablespoons butter
2 cloves garlic, minced
1 1/2 pounds chicken, cooked and cut into 1-inch chunks
1 can (7 3/4 ounces) pitted whole black ripe olives, drained

1 tablespoon dried basil
1 teaspoon salt
1/2 teaspoon black pepper
2 tablespoons cream
1/2 cup grated Parmesan or Romano cheese
4 slices bacon, cooked crisp and crumbled

Bring 2 inches of water to a boil in a large soup pot over a medium flame.

Add the cabbage strips and cook, covered, for 8 minutes, until soft.

Drain the cabbage in a colander and rinse under cold running water to prevent additional cooking. Place a bowl under the colander and set to one side.

In a large skillet, over low-medium heat, warm the butter until it begins to bubble (not brown). Reduce heat to low. Add the garlic and sauté, stirring continuously for 3 minutes.

Stir in the chicken chunks, olives, basil, salt, and pepper. Mix well and heat thoroughly. Reduce heat and slowly add the cream, stirring constantly for 1 minute.

Remove the chicken mixture from the stove and cover it to retain heat.

Place the cooked, drained cabbage into a large serving bowl. Add the chicken mixture and toss well. Add the Parmesan or Romano cheese and bacon, tossing once again to distribute flavors evenly.

Serve immediately.

Tuscan Marinade

PREP TIME: 7 minutes

COOK TIME: none

SERVINGS: 4

CARBS PER SERVING: 3 grams

We make enough of this marinade for two days, but it never lasts that long.

3/4 cup olive oil
2 cloves garlic, pressed
1/4 cup chopped fresh basil
(or 2 teaspoons dried basil)
1 teaspoon dried oregano
5 tablespoons lemon juice
Ground black pepper, as desired
2 stalks celery, cut into sticks (about 3 inches long)

2/3 cup sliced mushrooms
1 green bell pepper, cut into 1/2-inch strips
1/2 cucumber, peeled and sliced
1/8 head cauliflower, florets only
12 pitted whole olives, green or black ripe, drained

In a 12-ounce screw-top jar, combine the olive oil, garlic, basil, oregano, lemon juice and pepper as desired. Cover and shake well.

In a shallow bowl, combine the remaining ingredients, add the dressing, and toss to coat thoroughly. Cover and refrigerate overnight so that flavors penetrate and blend.

Drain and serve cold.

Anytime Antipasto

PREP TIME: 10 minutes
COOK TIME: none

SERVINGS: 4
CARBS PER SERVING: 4 grams

The secret of a good life is to build on what you've learned along the way. The secret of good cooking is the same. Combine two of your favorite recipes, add some extra goodies, and you can come up with an appetizer/snack that will surprise and delight you. Here's one of ours.

8 spinach leaves, washed and patted dry
4 slices provolone, rolled, seam side down
4 ounces mozzarella cheese, cut into 1-inch cubes
8 slices Bronx Salami (page 172)
4 radishes, cleaned and trimmed
8 pitted whole black ripe olives, drained

8 pitted whole green olives, drained
1/8 tomato (optional)
2 eggs, hard-boiled, peeled and halved
2 cups Tuscan Marinade (page 174)
   Grated Parmesan or Romano cheese, as desired
   Lemon wedges

Arrange 2 of the spinach leaves on each of 4 small serving plates.

Divide the remaining ingredients except the cheese and lemon among the 4 dishes, arranging them to please the eye.

Garnish with grated Parmesan or Romano as desired and the lemon wedges.

Serve cold.

Scallops Porta Rosa

PREP TIME: 13 minutes

COOK TIME: 15 minutes

SERVINGS: 4

CARBS PER SERVING: 1 gram

The finest Napa Valley restaurants serve seafood dishes that reflect the best in European cuisine. This recipe is inspired by their unique use of simple ingredients to bring about a surprisingly sophisticated flavor.

1/2 stick butter
1 clove garlic, pressed
3 scallions, diced
1 pound sea scallops, cleaned and patted dry with paper towels

Salt and pepper, as desired
1/4 cup chopped fresh parsley
1/3 cup heavy whipping cream
Grated Parmesan or Romano cheese, as desired

Warm the butter to the bubbling (not browning) point in a large saucepan over a medium flame. Reduce the heat to low and add the garlic and scallions. Cook, stirring often, for 3 minutes.

Add the scallops, stirring to coat well.

Cook the scallops, stirring constantly, over a medium flame for 5 to 8 minutes, until all sides have been exposed to the heat and the scallops are cooked through and completely opaque.

Add salt and pepper as desired.

Remove from heat. Add the parsley. Mix well.

Add the cream, toss well, and return to low heat for 1 minute to warm the mixture.

Top with grated Parmesan or Romano cheese as desired.

Serve immediately.

Crossbow Terrine

PREP TIME: 15 minutes
COOK TIME: 1 hour

SERVINGS: 4
CARBS PER SERVING: 2 grams

Each year in the Italian towns of Gubbio and Sansepolcro contestants challenge each other in a crossbow competition. The first contest was held in 1461, on the 17th of May, and a contest has been held on that date ever since. From what we've been told, this terrine might well have been served at that first match, as it is at today's.

1 pound sausage patties, fully cooked (or our Freedom Sausage, page 23, fully cooked), about 9 patties	2 teaspoons dried basil
	2 eggs, beaten
	Salt, pepper, and hot sauce, as desired
2 tablespoons olive oil	1/2 pound chicken breast slices, boneless and skinless, 1/4 to 1/2 inch thick
1/4 cup chopped onion	
1/2 teaspoon dried thyme	
1/4 teaspoon dried rosemary	

Preheat the oven to 375°F.

Divide the total number of sausage patties into thirds (about 3 patties to a third). Crumble one third of the patties, leaving the remaining two thirds whole. Put aside.

Heat the olive oil in a large skillet over a medium flame until hot (but not smoking). Add the onion and sauté for 5 minutes, until browned, stirring often to prevent sticking. Add the thyme, rosemary, and basil. Stir. Remove from heat, add the eggs, crumbled sausage patties, and salt, pepper, and hot sauce as desired. Mix well.

In a 9 × 5-inch loaf pan, lay down two rows of whole sausage patties, or enough to cover the entire bottom of the pan with no empty spaces.

Lay down alternate layers of chicken breast slices and sausage mixture, starting with chicken and ending with sausage mixture.

Bake for 1 hour. Remove the loaf pan and tilt carefully to drain off all fat.

Cut the terrine crossways into eight slices. Remove each slice with a pie server or small spatula and serve warm.

Classic Pesto

PREP TIME: 12 minutes **SERVINGS:** 4 (½ cup each)
COOK TIME: none **CARBS PER SERVING:** 3 grams (including pine nuts)

In the town of Te Anau, in the southernmost part of the South Island of New Zealand, we came across a cave filled with tens of thousands of glowworms. Though it was daytime outside, within the cave the little glowworms shone like stars against the perfectly black walls. That night, we ate pesto under the real stars in Te Anau's only Italian café. We were speechless during most of the meal, staring up at the sky that reminded us of the miracle of natural beauty we'd seen that day and still held in our hearts. Later we recaptured the feeling with this recipe.

½ cup grated Parmesan or Romano cheese
2 cloves garlic, pressed
½ cup olive oil (plus more if needed)
2 cups fresh basil leaves, washed and patted dry

¼ cup fresh parsley leaves, washed and patted dry with paper towels
2 tablespoons dried pignolias (pine nuts), optional

Combine all the ingredients in a food processor. Process until the pesto achieves the consistency of a thick, rich paste.

Add additional olive oil, as needed, 1 tablespoon at a time, to thin the pesto.

Toss with freshly boiled cabbage "pasta" (see Chicken Parmesan Romana, page 173) or use as a spread on meat, fish, or poultry before baking.

The pesto is also excellent as a dip for cucumber slices, raw cauliflower, or mushroom caps.

Scaloppine Palermo

PREP TIME: 11 minutes
COOK TIME: 30 minutes

SERVINGS: 4
CARBS PER SERVING: 2 grams

Near the Piazza Marina in the coastal town of Palermo, Sicily, the menus and recipes have remained unchanged for centuries. This recipe reflects the subtle combination of tastes that made us fall in love with the "flavor" of the city.

2 tablespoons butter
2 tablespoons olive oil
3 cloves garlic, minced
2 tablespoons paprika (hot or sweet)
1 tablespoon dried basil
1 teaspoon dried rosemary
3 green bell peppers, cut into 1/2-inch strips
6 mushrooms, sliced

1 pound veal, sliced thin (as for minute steak) and cut into 1/2-inch strips
1/4 cup chicken stock (or our Classic Chicken Stock, page 66)
1/4 cup lime juice
1/4 cup diced tomato
Salt and pepper, as desired

Heat the butter in a large skillet over a moderate flame until melted.

Add the oil and garlic. Sauté for about 2 minutes, stirring often.

Add the paprika, basil, rosemary, green peppers, and mushrooms. Stirring often, sauté until the peppers soften slightly (about 3 minutes) and the mushrooms release their liquid.

Move the garlic, peppers, and mushrooms to the sides of the pan and add the veal strips.

Sauté the veal strips, stirring often, so that all sides of the strips make contact with the hot surface and the meat is browned and thoroughly cooked (about 10 minutes).

Mix in the chicken stock, lime juice, and tomato, and simmer on low heat for 10 minutes.

Add salt and pepper, as desired.

Serve warm.

Spinach Lasagna

PREP TIME: 15 minutes

COOK TIME: 45 minutes

SERVINGS: 6

CARBS PER SERVING: 3 grams

Richard: *It was my birthday, the day before Rachael's, and I was craving lasagna. Rachael made this spinach version for me and, in a last flash of artistry, stuck candles in it. Once we removed the candles and the dripped wax, we enjoyed this dish for both my birthday and hers.*

For Layer #1

1/2 cup sour cream
2 eggs
1 package (10 ounces) frozen spinach, thawed and squeezed free of liquid

1 pound sausage patties, fully cooked and quartered (or our Freedom Sausage, page 23, fully cooked and quartered)

For Layer #2

8 ounces ricotta cheese
1 egg
1/2 cup grated mozzarella cheese

1 package (10 ounces) frozen spinach, drained and squeezed free of liquid

Topping

1/2 cup grated mozzarella cheese

Create the first layer by combining the sour cream and 2 eggs in a mixing bowl. Beat until smooth.

Add spinach and sausage and blend with a fork until well distributed.

Place about half of the mixture in a lasagna pan (9 × 12 inches) to form a bottom layer.

Preheat the oven to 375°F.

In a medium-size bowl, combine the ingredients for Layer #2. Spread all the mixture as a single layer over the sausage layer.

(continued)

Gently spread the remainder of the sausage mixture over Layer #2 to form a top layer.

Bake for 30 minutes.

Remove from the oven and top evenly with the grated mozzarella.

Return to the oven for an additional 15 minutes, until the topping begins to bubble and turns golden brown.

JAPANESE
JEWELS

Fundamental Fish Stock

PREP TIME: 20 minutes
COOK TIME: 75 minutes

SERVINGS: 4 (1 cup each)
CARBS PER SERVING: 1 gram

An essential for many dishes and delicious all by itself as a hearty broth.

1/2 cup minced onion
2 stalks celery, chopped
1/4 stick butter
2 tablespoons fresh lemon juice
1/4 cup dry white wine (optional)
1 tablespoon soy sauce

Dash of ground black pepper
4 cups chicken stock (or our Classic Chicken Stock, page 66)
1 pound mild fish (flounder, sole, mahimahi, monkfish, etc.), carefully deboned and cut into 1-inch chunks

In a medium-size saucepan over a medium flame, cook the onion and celery in the butter, stirring, until the onion becomes transparent.

Add the lemon juice, wine, soy sauce, and pepper, stirring constantly. Cook until the wine is reduced by half (about 15 minutes), then add the stock and fish chunks.

Bring to a boil, lower heat, and simmer covered, for 30 minutes, stirring occasionally. Remove cover and continue to simmer for another 30 minutes. Remove from heat and allow to cool enough to handle.

Then process small batches in a blender or food processor, until all solids disappear into the stock.

Use at once or freeze in premeasured packages until needed.

Besford's Blessed Seaweed Soup

PREP TIME: 4 minutes
COOK TIME: 5 minutes

SERVINGS: 4
CARBS PER SERVING: 1 gram

Richard: *The Hotel Mira Costa at Tokyo Disney Resort is breathtakingly beautiful and superbly well managed. Unfortunately, Rachael had such a bad cold when we were there that she couldn't enjoy anything. The manager of the hotel, Charles Besford, hearing of her illness, took time to personally arrange to send her all the seaweed soup she wanted, along with special Japanese wipes to cool her fevered brow. Within a day, Rachael's temperature was back to normal, the aches had subsided, and our vacation for two was rescued from the ashes. Here's our version of that seaweed lifesaver.*

4 cups fish stock (or our Fundamental Fish Stock, page 185)
1/2 cup thinly sliced scallions
1 block (about 4 × 4 inches) tofu*, firm, drained and cut in 1-inch cubes

2 cups cooked and shredded chicken (optional)
4 sheets (4 × 4 inches each) nori seaweed, pre-roasted and ready to eat (or 1/4 cup thinly sliced red radishes)

In a medium-size saucepan over a medium flame, heat the fish stock and scallions until near boiling (about 3 minutes). Stir occasionally.

Reduce heat to low.

Add the tofu cubes and shredded chicken. Allow to warm but not boil (about 2 minutes).

Crumble the seaweed, or float red radish slices, on top and serve warm.

*See page 6 for our Easy but Essential Tofu Tip.

Tanaka-san Shrimp Salad

PREP TIME: 13 minutes

COOK TIME: none

SERVINGS: 4

CARBS PER SERVING: 2 grams

We were strangers in Japan, but Toshio Tanaka and his wife, Etsuko, made us feel like welcome guests. Tanaka-san gave up his day off so that he could show us the magnificent shrines and temples of Kamakura. At the end of the day, we were filled with the power of this spiritual experience. A heavy American meal would have felt wrong, so the world's best tour guide (and friend) brought us to a quiet Japanese restaurant where we were served a delicate shrimp dish. Here's our interpretation of the dish that nourished both body and soul.

Dressing Ingredients

1/2 cup lime juice

2 tablespoons olive oil

4 scallions, split lengthwise
   down the middle, in halves

1/4 teaspoon prepared wasabi
   (or 1 tablespoon white
   prepared horseradish)

4 anchovies, mashed to paste

Salad Base

20 large shrimp, cooked,
   shelled, and deveined

1 head lettuce (romaine
   preferred), washed,
   dried, and cut into 1-inch
   strips

3/4 cup mint leaves,
   washed, dried, and cut
   into thin strips

1/2 cup fresh basil leaves,
   cut into thin strips

1 hard-boiled egg, shelled
   and sliced

1 cup alfalfa sprouts
   (optional)

Combine all the dressing ingredients in a large salad bowl. Whisk well.

Split each shrimp down the middle. Toss all the shrimp with the dressing.

(continued)

Place in the refrigerator for 30 minutes. Remove shrimp and scallion halves and place them on a separate plate.

Transfer the lettuce, mint, and basil leaves to the salad bowl and toss well with the dressing.

Divide the lettuce mixture among four salad bowls and top with the split shrimp and scallion halves.

Garnish with slices of hard-boiled egg and alfalfa sprouts, and drizzle with any dressing remaining in the bottom of the mixing bowl.

Chiba Pork Roast

PREP TIME: 12 minutes

COOK TIME: 2 hours or more

SERVINGS: 6

CARBS PER SERVING: 3 grams

In Japan, the portions of meat and fish dishes are tiny (almost like hors d'oeuvres) by American standards. When our Japanese hosts noticed that we were used to large portions of protein, but that we were restraining ourselves out of consideration for others, a luscious pork roast suddenly appeared as part of the menu.

2 pounds loin of pork roast
4 tablespoons olive oil
2 tablespoons soy sauce
2 tablespoons garlic powder
1/2 teaspoon dried rosemary
1/2 teaspoon dried thyme

1/2 cup grated daikon (optional)
1 cup spinach, washed and shredded
3/4 cup sliced mushrooms (or 2 cups whole mushrooms)

Preheat the oven to 350°F.

Place the pork roast on a rack in a deep roasting pan, fat side up. Fill the bottom of the pan with water to the 1 1/2-inch level (so that pork on the rack does not touch the water in the pan). Insert a meat thermometer in the thickest portion of the roast, away from any bone.

Wash your hands thoroughly.

Brush the oil on all exposed surfaces of the pork roast, including fat.

Brush the soy sauce on all exposed surfaces of the pork roast, including fat.

In a small bowl mix together the garlic powder, rosemary, and thyme. Sprinkle the herb mixture over all exposed surfaces of the pork roast, including fat.

Place the roasting pan in the oven, maintaining the water level at 1 inch or more throughout the roasting process. Baste the roast with juices from the bottom of the pan at least once every half hour.

Roast for at least 45 minutes *for each pound* of meat, or until a meat thermometer registers well done for pork.

Fifteen minutes prior to the roast being done, add the grated daikon, shredded raw spinach, and mushrooms to the gravy at the bottom of the roasting pan.

(continued)

When the pork is cooked through and the ideal internal temperature of 170°F has been reached, remove the pan from the oven. Allow the roast to rest on the rack and the vegetables to remain in the au jus gravy. The roast may be carved after resting for 7 minutes.

Serve the vegetables warm with the sliced roast.

Marinated Squid

PREP TIME: 12 minutes
COOK TIME: 13 minutes

SERVINGS: 4
CARBS PER SERVING: 3 grams

If you like calamari, you'll love this authentic Japanese dish.

1/2 cup olive oil
2 tablespoons soy sauce
4 scallions, finely chopped
2 teaspoons garlic, pressed
1/4 teaspoon prepared wasabi
(or 1 tablespoon white
prepared horseradish)

1 teaspoon peeled and finely
grated fresh ginger root
1/4 cup lime juice
1 pound squid, cleaned,
bodies and tentacles left
whole

In a small saucepan, mix the olive oil, soy sauce, scallions, garlic, wasabi, ginger root, and lime juice, whisking to combine as well as possible.

Warm, uncovered, over a low heat (do not bring to a boil).

Remove the marinade from the heat and transfer it to a large bowl. Allow it to cool to lukewarm.

Add the squid and marinate, covered, overnight in the refrigerator, mixing occasionally to ensure that all surfaces of the squid are covered with marinade.

When you're ready to cook the squid, drain and discard the marinade. Heat a wok (or large skillet) over a medium flame and add the squid. Stir-fry for 6 to 7 minutes, until the squid is cooked and opaque throughout. (Marinade on the surface of the squid will provide enough oil to stir-fry.)

Serve immediately.

Daikon Salad

PREP TIME: 11 minutes
COOK TIME: none

SERVINGS: 4
CARBS PER SERVING: 2 grams

This dish is traditionally made with arame, *a Japanese sea vegetable. Although we searched for a substitute for two years, we found no American equivalent. Nothing came close. The recent appearance of daikon, also known as Japanese radish, in many American supermarkets has more than solved the problem. Now we can enjoy this super salad whenever we want.*

Salad Base

3 cups grated daikon
1 cup julienne green bell
   pepper

2 stalks celery, julienne
2 scallions, sliced thin

Dressing Ingredients

6 tablespoons olive oil
2 teaspoons sesame oil
1 clove garlic, minced
1/2 teaspoon peeled and grated
   fresh ginger root

1 teaspoon white vinegar (or
   lemon juice)
1/2 teaspoon soy sauce
4 anchovies, mashed
   (optional)

In a large salad bowl, combine all the salad ingredients and toss well to mix evenly. Refrigerate the salad while you prepare the dressing.

In a 12-ounce screw-top jar, combine all the dressing ingredients. Cover and shake very well.

Drizzle the dressing over the salad ingredients and toss well.

Serve immediately.

VARIATION

Sliced, hard-boiled eggs placed on top of this salad soak up and complement the tangy dressing.

Mock Seaweed Soup

PREP TIME: 12 minutes

COOK TIME: 12 minutes

SERVINGS: 4

CARBS PER SERVING: 3 grams

Tokyo Bay is filled with dozens of exciting places to spend your yen and your carbs. The waiter informed us that the seaweed soup was on the house (we wouldn't have ordered it ourselves) and . . . we loved it! All attempts to make it at home, however, were disastrous—way too salty. Here's a mocked-up version that's far more suited to our American tastes.

1 tablespoon butter

1 teaspoon sesame oil

1 stalk celery, chopped

2 scallions, chopped

1 cup sliced mushrooms

1 teaspoon peeled, thinly sliced fresh ginger root

1 block (about 4 × 4 inches) tofu*, firm, drained and cut into 1-inch cubes

4 cups chicken stock (or our Classic Chicken Stock, page 66)

2 cups fresh spinach, washed and shredded

Soy sauce and ground white pepper, as desired

Heat the butter and sesame oil together in a large skillet over a medium flame until warm but not bubbling, Add the celery, scallions, mushrooms, and ginger root. Sauté until softened, about 5 minutes, stirring often.

Reduce heat to low. Add the tofu and toss thoroughly with the other ingredients. Warm through for 3 to 4 minutes, stirring often to baste the tofu. Remove the skillet from the heat and set it aside.

In a large soup pot, heat the chicken stock until stock at the pan's edges begins to bubble (but does not come to a full boil).

Add the spinach. Reduce the heat to low and cook until the spinach is wilted, about 3 minutes. Turn off the heat and cover the pot, leaving it on the burner to keep it warm.

Using a slotted spatula, lift the tofu and vegetables from the skillet, allowing all the butter and oil to drain off, and transfer the tofu and vegetables to the soup stock.

Add soy sauce and ground white pepper, as desired.

Mix well and serve immediately.

*See page 6 for our Easy but Essential Tofu Tip.

Asian Chicken Nuggets

PREP TIME: 7 minutes
COOK TIME: 45 minutes

SERVINGS: 6
CARBS PER SERVING: 1 gram

The buffet at the Oceano restaurant at Hotel Mira Costa at Tokyo Disney Resort seems to go on forever. The chefs include recipes from around the world, insuring that each person finds both familiar and new dishes at the same meal. The chicken dish that inspired this recipe combined flavors from at least three Asian countries in a perfect blend that both kids and adults loved!

3 cups olive oil	1 teaspoon dried basil
2 tablespoons soy oil	1 teaspoon ground rosemary
3 cloves garlic, minced	1/2 teaspoon crushed red
1/4 cup diced onion	pepper
1 tablespoon peeled and grated fresh ginger root	2 pounds chicken breasts, boned and skinned, cut into
1 tablespoon curry powder	1-inch chunks
1 teaspoon ground coriander	Nonstick cooking spray

In a large bowl, combine the olive oil, soy sauce, garlic, onion, ginger root, curry powder, coriander, basil, rosemary, and red pepper to form a marinade. Whisk together well.

Add the chicken chunks to the marinade. Cover and refrigerate overnight.

Immediately prior to cooking, preheat the oven to 375°F.

Remove the chicken chunks from the marinade and discard the marinade.

Spray a baking sheet with nonstick cooking spray, and place the chicken nuggets on the baking sheet.

Bake for 45 minutes, until cooked throughout, turning often with a spatula to expose all surfaces to heat. Nuggets will be crispy and brown when they're done.

Serve the nuggets when they are cool enough to handle. Spear each one with a toothpick and dunk them in any low-carb dip. Our Instant Onion Dip, page 225, is especially good.

Grab-and-Go Low-Carb Sushi

PREP TIME: 10 minutes
COOK TIME: 6 to 8 minutes

SERVINGS: 8 (3 sushi each)
CARBS PER SERVING: 0 to 1 gram

Sushi lovers don't have to give up sushi just because they're on low-carb diets. This no-rice alternative allows you to enjoy your favorite flavors and textures without the carbs. One note of caution, however: because we are not using sticky rice or rice wine vinegar, the cauliflower-filled sushi does not stick together well, and can be a mess to eat. You can conquer that problem by using bigger pieces of roasted nori (Japanese seaweed, found in many supermarkets) as a "pocket" to enfold and secure your sushi package. You might want to experiment until you find the method of delivery that works best for you. In any case, you'll find the taste well worth the effort.

Riced Cauliflower (use in sushi as low-carb substitute for rice)

1 head cauliflower, florets only

For Sushi Wrapping

6 sheets (4 × 4 inches each) roasted nori (seaweed), cut into quarters

For Sushi Filling

Choice of *cooked* bits of:
squid
shrimp
salmon roe
salmon

grilled eel
omelet
(For safety concerns, use fully cooked seafood and eggs only.)

For Garnish (as desired)

Thin cucumber slices
Grated ginger

Very thin slices of garlic or scallion
Bits of cilantro

(continued)

For Spice (as desired)

Prepared wasabi   Soy sauce
Hot sauce

To Prepare the Riced Cauliflower:

In a large saucepan, over high heat, bring 1¹/₂ inches of water to a boil. Add the cauliflower florets and boil for 4 minutes exactly. Remove from heat, drain the florets in a colander, and rinse them under cold running water to stop cooking immediately. When the florets are cool enough to handle easily, transfer them to a large cutting board.

Using a nonserrated knife, repeatedly chop the florets until the cauliflower takes on a "riced" texture (tiny, non-mushy bits). Using a spatula, carefully scrape the riced cauliflower into a medium-size bowl and put aside, uncovered and at room temperature, to be used immediately in the making of the sushi.

To Assemble Sushi:

Spoon 1 or 2 rounded tablespoons of riced cauliflower into the center of a section of nori, folding it up around the edges to form a pocket.

Make a deep indentation in the middle of the cauliflower using your little finger.

Fill the indentation with a sushi filling of your choice, including cooked bits of squid, shrimp, salmon roe, salmon, grilled eel, omelet, or any other *cooked* filling you desire.

Garnish with any of the following: thin cucumber slices, grated ginger, very thin slices of garlic or scallion, or bits of cilantro.

Serve with prepared wasabi, hot sauce, and soy sauce on the side.

Delicate Crab Sandwiches

PREP TIME: 15 minutes
COOK TIME: none

SERVINGS: 4 (5 tiny sandwiches per serving)
CARBS PER SERVING: 1 gram

After a long morning of white-water rafting Japanese style, we expected a hearty lunch. We assumed that the tiny hors d'oeuvres we were served were only the first course. We soon realized, however, that they were the whole meal, and that, though light, they were surprisingly filling. Once we'd enjoyed them to our heart's content, we were more than ready to face an afternoon of countless calls from our rafting guide to "mai-kogi" (forward paddle) and "skah-mah-tae" (hold on)!

1 pound crabmeat, freshly cooked or canned, drained and patted dry with paper towels
1 teaspoon dried onion flakes

1 teaspoon soy sauce
1/2 teaspoon parsley flakes
2 teaspoons cream cheese
2 cucumbers, thinly sliced, patted dry with paper towels

Put the crabmeat, onion flakes, soy sauce, parsley flakes, and cream cheese in a food processor. Process to a thick paste (retaining some small chunks of crabmeat).

Spread the crabmeat paste onto half of the cucumber slices. Top each little crabmeat mound with a second cucumber slice to make sandwiches.

Yellow Dragon Tofu

PREP TIME: 13 minutes
COOK TIME: 4 minutes

SERVINGS: 4
CARBS PER SERVING: 2 grams

We had spent a fun day exploring the great attractions along the Tokyo-to-Chiba subway line. Tired and hungry, but victorious, we stopped in a little restaurant that sported a yellow dragon on its sign. We'll never find the restaurant again and we never discovered what gave this dish its smoky flavor (we've had to improvise a lot here), but we'll never forget the sweet satisfaction of having navigated the city on our own, despite our inability to speak Japanese, or the delicious reward we happened upon.

1 tablespoon olive oil
2 blocks (about 4 × 4 inches each), tofu*, firm, drained and cut into 1-inch cubes
1/2 cup diced celery
1/2 cup green beans (or wax or snap beans), trimmed

2 tablespoons soy sauce
2 cloves garlic, minced
1/2 teaspoon dried thyme
6 slices bacon, cooked crisp and crumbled
2 tablespoons lime juice

In a medium-size skillet combine the olive oil, tofu, celery, green beans, soy sauce, garlic, and thyme. Heat over a medium flame, careful of sputtering, until the oil is warm (but not smoking), stirring the tofu and green beans often to coat (about 4 minutes).

Remove from heat. Add the bacon and stir well.

Turn onto a plate and drizzle with lime juice.

Serve immediately.

*See page 6 for our Easy but Essential Tofu Tip.

Kyoto Marinated Steak Strips

PREP TIME: 5 minutes

COOK TIME: 20 to 25 minutes

SERVINGS: 4

CARBS PER SERVING: 1 gram

A few years ago, the ingredients in this recipe could be found only in Asian markets. Today, with the widespread interest in Japanese cuisine, you'll probably find miso (soybean paste) and wasabi in the spice aisle or Asian food section of your local supermarket. You might not be accustomed to cooking with these ingredients, but once you try, you'll find that their special flavors zip up any meat, poultry, or seafood dish.

1/8 cup miso (soybean paste)

1/4 cup dry white wine (or 2 tablespoons lemon juice and 1/4 cup beef stock, or our Classic Beef Stock, page 67)

1/4 teaspoon prepared wasabi (or 1 tablespoon white prepared horseradish)

2 cloves garlic, sliced thin

1 tablespoon white vinegar

1 pound strip steak, trimmed, and cut into 1-inch-wide strips

6 leaves spinach, washed, dried, and refrigerated (optional)

Combine the miso, wine, prepared wasabi, garlic, and vinegar in a large bowl. Whisk together well.

Add the steak strips. Cover the bowl and marinate the meat in the refrigerator for 2 hours, tossing every 15 minutes to ensure that all surfaces are exposed to the marinade.

Drain the meat and discard the marinade.

Over a medium-high flame, in a wok or medium-size nonstick skillet, stir-fry the meat, browning all its surfaces. The meat will retain enough oil from the marinade to allow you to stir-fry it without adding more oil.

Reduce the flame to medium and continue cooking and stirring until the meat is thoroughly cooked (15 to 20 minutes).

Serve the steak warm on a bed of cool, crisp spinach leaves.

Osaka Hot and Sour Mushrooms

PREP TIME: 8 minutes

COOK TIME: 5 minutes

SERVINGS: 6

CARBS PER SERVING: 2 grams

The most striking difference between Japanese and American cuisine is the remarkably small servings that are considered customary in Japan. When we were served this dish at an international benefit luncheon we thought it was the first course, but along with some sautéed spinach, it constituted the entire meal. Still, we all enjoyed and appreciated it, and back home, we serve our version of it as an hors d'oeuvre.

2 cups chicken stock (or our Classic Chicken Stock, page 66)
1/4 cup lime juice (or lemon juice)
1 tablespoon lime zest (or lemon zest)
2 cloves garlic, minced
1 stalk celery, chopped
1 teaspoon dried basil

1/2 teaspoon dried thyme
Prepared wasabi (or white prepared horseradish, crushed red pepper, or hot sauce), as desired
2 teaspoons soy sauce
1 block (about 4 × 4 inches) tofu*, firm, drained and cut into 1-inch cubes
1 pound mushroom caps
2 sheets (2 × 2 inches each) nori seaweed, pre-roasted and cut in quarters
Wooden toothpicks

Combine the chicken stock, juice, zest, garlic, chopped celery, basil, thyme, wasabi as desired, soy sauce, and tofu in a large soup pot over a low flame.

Warm the mixture but do not bring to a boil, stirring often but gently to keep the tofu cubes intact.

Remove the pot from the heat and allow to cool to room temperature.

Pour it into a large bowl and marinate for 6 to 8 hours in the refrigerator.

(continued)

*See page 6 for our Easy but Essential Tofu Tip.

Remove the bowl from the refrigerator and strain, leaving behind only the tofu and mushrooms.

To assemble hors d'oeuvres, line each inverted mushroom cap with 1 tiny square of roasted nori. Pierce each tofu cube with a toothpick, then stick it into one of the inverted mushroom caps.

Serve cold, being careful to tell people to remove all toothpicks before eating.

NON-MEAT CUISINE

Classic Tofu Burgers

PREP TIME: 13 minutes

COOK TIME: 40 minutes

SERVINGS: 3

CARBS PER SERVING: 4 grams

Rachael: *While in school, I was a vegetarian for two years, out of both financial and ethical concerns. There was no kitchen in my one-room apartment, only a hot plate and an electric toaster, but I learned to cook low-carb vegetarian dishes that smelled and tasted so good, they made my classmates jealous. These "burgers" were a favorite I could always count on.*

1 tablespoon butter
1 cup sliced mushrooms
3 tablespoons olive oil
2 cloves garlic, crushed
1/2 green bell pepper, finely minced
2 stalks celery, finely chopped
1 block (about 4 × 4 inches)

tofu*, extra firm, drained and mashed
2 eggs
1 teaspoon dried basil
1/2 cup grated cheese (cheddar or American)
Salt, pepper, cayenne, and paprika, as desired

Preheat the oven to 350°F.

Heat the butter in a medium-size skillet over a medium flame.

Add the mushroom slices and sauté, stirring often, until golden brown (about 4 minutes).

Remove the skillet from the heat. Using a slotted spatula, transfer the mushroom slices to a small bowl. Set aside. Discard the mushroom drippings from the skillet.

Heat 2 tablespoons of the olive oil in the skillet. Add the garlic, green pepper, and celery. Mix well and sauté over medium heat, stirring often, for 2 minutes or until the green pepper and celery soften.

Remove the pan from the heat and, using a slotted spatula, transfer the mixture to a medium-size bowl. Add the tofu, eggs, basil, and cheese. Mix thoroughly, adding salt, pepper, cayenne, and paprika as desired. Put aside.

Use the remaining tablespoon of olive oil to coat a baking sheet.

Shape the tofu mixture into three 3-inch patties and place them on the greased baking sheet.

(continued)

*See page 6 for our Easy but Essential Tofu Tip.

Place the baking sheet in the oven and bake the patties for 25 to 30 minutes, or until the "burgers" are well cooked throughout and browned.

About 5 minutes before the "burgers" are finished, transfer the mushroom slices to the baking sheet around the "burgers" and return the sheet to the oven.

Serve the "burgers" warm, topped with mushroom slices, and accompanied by our Tofu Crisps (page 103) or fresh low-carb vegetables.

Low-Carb Lasagna

PREP TIME: 15 minutes
COOK TIME: 30 to 35 minutes

SERVINGS: 8
CARBS PER SERVING: 4 grams

*This recipe is very special to us. It was born out of an unwilling-
ness to give up, from a score of tries and retries until we got it right.
The thin wedges of portobello mushroom act as an excellent substitute for the pasta and can be used in place of meat in a host of other
low-carb recipes.*

2 tablespoons olive oil

Filling

3 cups ricotta cheese
4 tablespoons grated
   Parmesan or Romano
   cheese
1/4 teaspoon dried basil

1 teaspoon dried oregano
1/2 tablespoon parsley flakes
1/2 teaspoon garlic powder
   Salt and pepper, as desired

Layers

4 portobello mushrooms,
   sliced in half crosswise, then
   quartered into wedges, so
   that each mushroom yields
   8 thin wedges

1 package (10 ounces) frozen
   spinach, thawed and
   squeezed free of liquid
6 ounces cooked chicken,
   pork, or steak, sliced thin
   (optional)
1 1/2 cups shredded mozzarella
   cheese

Preheat the oven to 350°F.

Oil a lasagna pan and gather all the ingredients before beginning
the assembly of the lasagna.

Place the filling ingredients in a medium-size mixing bowl and stir
well. Put aside.

Arrange the mushroom wedges as a first layer on the bottom of the
lasagna pan. Cover them with a thin layer of spinach, then some of

(continued)

the cooked meat or chicken (optional), and finally a layer of mozzarella (about one third of each).

Lay down another layer of mushroom wedges. Add half the cheese filling, spreading it evenly over the mushrooms. Repeat another layer of spinach, followed by cooked meat or chicken (again, optional) and mozzarella (another third of each).

Add a last layer of thin mushroom wedges. Add the rest of the cheese filling, followed by the rest of the spinach, cooked meat or chicken, and finishing with mozzarella.

Bake the lasagna for 30 to 35 minutes, until the top is golden and bubbly. Remove the dish from the oven and allow the lasagna to cool to warm before serving.

Spicy (or Mild)
Vegetarian Stir-Fry

PREP TIME: 5 minutes

COOK TIME: 3 to 4 minutes

SERVINGS: 2

CARBS PER SERVING: 5 grams

We whip this dish up whenever we want something exciting. We add whatever leftovers we think will work and, somehow, they always do!

1 block (about 4 × 4 inches) tofu*, firm, drained and cut into 1-inch cubes
1 teaspoon soy sauce
2 teaspoons sesame oil
2 tablespoon peanut oil
1/2 cup diced green bell pepper

1/2 cup chopped celery
1 tablespoon capers
2 dried red chili peppers, for spicy flavor (less, as desired, for milder taste)
3 cups shredded raw cabbage (optional)

Place the tofu cubes in a medium-size bowl. Add the soy sauce and gently mix to distribute. Put aside.

In a separate medium-size bowl, combine all the other ingredients except cabbage. Whisk well and pour over the tofu cubes, tossing gently to ensure full coverage but without breaking the cubes.

Transfer the mixture to a medium-size skillet and heat over a low-medium flame until warmed but not simmering (3 to 4 minutes). Gently stir to ensure even heating. Using a fork, remove and discard the chili peppers.

Serve the tofu warm over shredded raw cabbage. Drizzle with pan drippings.

*See page 6 for our Easy but Essential Tofu Tip.

Mashed "Potatoes" (With All the Fixings)

PREP TIME: 10 minutes
COOK TIME: 25 minutes

SERVINGS: 4
CARBS PER SERVING: 2 to 5 grams
(depending on choice of fixings)

Makes you realize that it's the toppings you love best.

1 head cauliflower
3 ounces cream cheese, quartered and well softened

Salt and pepper, as desired
Paprika (hot or sweet) as garnish

All the Fixings

Grated cheddar cheese
Crisply cooked and crumbled bacon (optional)
Chopped chives

Chopped scallions
Dollop of sour cream
Butter

Quarter the cauliflower and cook it in 1 inch of boiling water in a medium-size stockpot or large saucepan, covered, for 5 minutes.

Drain well and set in the refrigerator to cool.

Transfer the cold cauliflower to a food processor and process until it forms pea-size bits, or chop it well in a chopping bowl.

Place the processed cauliflower into a medium-size bowl. Add the softened cream cheese quarters one at a time, mixing and mashing just a little after each addition, until a consistency of mashed potatoes is reached.

Add salt and pepper, as desired. Mix once more, gently but thoroughly.

Sprinkle with paprika and warm the mashed "potatoes" in a small, covered microwavable container, 2 minutes on low-medium setting, or bake in a 350°F oven, uncovered, for 20 minutes.

Top with any of your favorite low-carb choices: grated cheese, bacon bits (if desired), chives, scallions, sour cream, or butter.

Tofu Dijon Sauce

PREP TIME: 4 minutes
COOK TIME: none

SERVINGS: 4 (¼ cup each)
CARBS PER SERVING: 2 grams

This healthy and low-carb alternative for honey-mustard dressing will make you happy you're eating low-carb.

1 block (about 4 × 4 inches) tofu*, drained and quartered
6 tablespoons Dijon mustard
6 tablespoons olive oil

1 tablespoon white wine vinegar
2 cloves garlic, minced
3 drops chili oil (optional)

Combine all of the ingredients in a blender or food processor and purée until smooth.

Refrigerate for 2 to 4 hours and serve cold on cauliflower, asparagus, or green beans, or as a dip for low-carb raw vegetables, including mushrooms, celery, and cucumber slices. It's especially good with fresh green pepper wedges.

*See page 6 for our Easy but Essential Tofu Tip.

Tofu Western Melt

PREP TIME: 4 minutes
COOK TIME: 6 to 7 minutes

SERVINGS: 2
CARBS PER SERVING: 5 grams

A no-egg omelet that's great any time of the day (or night).

1 tablespoon olive oil
2 teaspoons finely chopped onion
4 mushrooms, sliced
1/4 cup diced green bell peppers
2 teaspoons finely diced fresh tomato
1 block (about 4 × 4 inches) tofu*, drained and cut into 1-inch squares

1/2 teaspoon dried basil
1/2 teaspoon paprika (hot or sweet)
Salt, white or black pepper, and cayenne, as desired
1 cup grated cheese (cheddar, American, Swiss, or Monterey Jack)

Heat the olive oil in a nonstick medium-size skillet over a medium flame and sauté the onions, mushrooms, peppers, and tomato until the onions begin to brown (3 minutes).

Add the tofu cubes and sauté 3 to 4 minutes, stirring gently with a nonstick spatula.

Turn the heat to low. Add the basil and paprika and salt, pepper, and cayenne as desired. Stir gently with the spatula once again.

Sprinkle with the cheese, cover with a tight-fitting lid, and remove from heat.

Serve warm once the cheese has melted (3 to 4 minutes).

*See page 6 for our Easy but Essential Tofu Tip.

Butter "Burgers"

PREP TIME: 5 minutes

COOK TIME: 8 to 10 minutes

SERVINGS: 4

CARBS PER SERVING: 4 grams

Good anytime for a meal or a snack but best when served freshly cooked and still warm.

1/2 stick butter, softened

1/2 teaspoon garlic powder

1/4 cup fresh parsley (or
    1 tablespoon dried parsley)

2 teaspoons finely diced
    onion

1/3 cup sliced mushrooms

1 tablespoon olive oil

4 vegetarian "burgers" (found
    in many supermarket
    freezers), thawed per
    package directions

1 lemon, quartered

Combine the butter, garlic powder, and parsley in a medium-size mixing bowl.

Wet your hands and shape the butter into 4 balls. Chill until solid.

In a medium-size skillet over a medium flame, cook the onions and mushrooms in olive oil until they turn a golden brown.

Add the vegetarian "burgers" and fry until browned on both sides (6 to 8 minutes in total) and cooked through.

With a slotted spatula, remove the "burgers," mushrooms, and bits of onions to a covered casserole dish.

Top each "burger" with a butter ball and cover until melted (2 minutes).

Sprinkle with lemon juice and serve.

Hearty Meatless Casserole

PREP TIME: 9 minutes
COOK TIME: 30 minutes

SERVINGS: 4
CARBS PER SERVING: 2 grams

The mushrooms in this dish give it a "meaty" flavor, the cheese provides protein, and it works well as a main dish or as an extra-special side dish.

1 tablespoon olive oil (or use nonstick cooking spray)
1 clove garlic, crushed
2 portobello mushrooms, sliced in half crosswise, then quartered into wedges, so that each mushroom yields 8 thin wedges
2 tablespoons butter
3 cups green beans (or wax or snap beans) that have been trimmed and cut into 2-inch sections

1 tablespoon dried basil
Salt, pepper, and cayenne, as desired
1 cup grated cheese (cheddar, American, Swiss, or Monterey Jack)
Paprika (hot or sweet)
Sour cream, as garnish (optional)

Preheat the oven to 375°F.

Oil a deep ovenproof casserole dish. Put aside.

Using a medium-size skillet, sauté the garlic and thin mushroom wedges in the butter for 3 to 4 minutes, turning occasionally.

When the mushroom wedges begin to turn golden brown, reduce heat to low-medium and remove the mushroom wedges with a slotted spatula, allowing pan drippings to remain in the skillet. Arrange half of the mushroom wedges on a plate and lay the other half in the bottom of the casserole dish so that they form a buttery base layer.

Place the green beans in the skillet. Sauté for 4 to 6 minutes in the remaining butter and garlic, stirring occasionally. Add more butter as needed to prevent sticking.

When the green beans begin to soften, remove the pan from the heat and transfer the beans to a medium-size bowl.

Add the basil and salt, pepper, and cayenne as desired. Toss well.

(continued)

Transfer half the green bean mixture to the casserole dish. Set aside the remainder.

Sprinkle half of the grated cheese onto the green bean mixture in the casserole dish and repeat layering with the remainder of the mushroom wedges, green bean mixture, and grated cheese, in that order.

Sprinkle paprika over the top layer of cheese and bake for 20 minutes, or until the cheese is bubbly.

Allow the casserole to cool a bit, cut into squares, and serve warm with a dollop of sour cream on the side.

Old-Fashioned "Chicken" Casserole

PREP TIME: 11 minutes

COOK TIME: 38 minutes

SERVINGS: 4

CARBS PER SERVING: 5 grams

Meat alternatives can be counted on to pick up the flavor of foods they are cooked in. The more you put into the sauce, the more you get out of the recipe. This "old-fashioned" dish brings the best of traditional cooking to a no-meat meal.

3 tablespoons olive oil

2 teaspoons chopped scallions

1 green bell pepper, chopped

6 celery stalks, finely chopped

2 teaspoons peeled and grated fresh ginger root

3 cloves garlic, crushed

8 vegetable protein "chicken" cutlets (found in many supermarket freezers), thawed per package directions

1½ cups sour cream

1 teaspoon dried dill

¼ cup water

Preheat the oven to 350°F.

Coat the bottom of a 2-quart ovenproof casserole dish with 1 tablespoon of the olive oil. Put aside.

Warm the remaining 2 tablespoons of olive oil in a large skillet over medium heat.

Add the scallions, peppers, celery, ginger, and garlic and sauté, stirring often, until the peppers and celery begin to soften (about 3 minutes).

Add the "chicken" cutlets to the skillet, stir gently, and sauté until the cutlets are warmed with the mixture (about 5 minutes).

Transfer the cutlets and vegetable mixture to the casserole dish. Set aside.

In a small bowl, combine the sour cream, dill, and water. Mix well.

Pour the sour cream mixture over the cutlets and bake for 30 minutes.

Feng Shui Curry

PREP TIME: 5 minutes
COOK TIME: none

SERVINGS: 2
CARBS PER SERVING: 4 grams

We used to think of curry as Indian cuisine, but we've discovered that the Japanese make some of the best curry dishes in the world. This unusual cold curry recipe brings together three Asian ingredients that balance perfectly; a sort of feng shui for your palate that is a wonderful light summer treat.

1 package (10 ounces) frozen spinach, thawed and squeezed free of liquid
1 cup light whipping cream
2 fresh red or green chili peppers*, seeded and quartered (or prepared wasabi, as desired)

1 block (about 4 × 4 inches) tofu†, firm, drained and cut into 1/2-inch cubes
1 clove garlic, minced
1 teaspoon curry powder
2 cups grated daikon

In a large bowl, combine the spinach, cream, chili peppers, tofu, garlic, and curry powder.

Toss the ingredients well but carefully to ensure blending of all flavors without breaking the tofu cubes. Refrigerate, covered, for 2 hours.

While the tofu is marinating, line two plates with grated daikon.

Using a slotted spatula, lift the spinach and tofu from the marinade and transfer them to the daikon-lined plates. Serve immediately.

Discard the remainder of the marinade, including the chili peppers.

*NOTE: When handling chili peppers, it's always a good idea to wear rubber or latex gloves. The pepper can burn and irritate your hands even if you are not aware of any tiny cuts or abrasions that may exist. Be certain not to touch your face or eyes or any other area that may be vulnerable to damage or irritation. Immediately wash knife, cutting surfaces, and gloves when finished.

†See page 6 for our Easy but Essential Tofu Tip.

Friday Night "Steak"

PREP TIME: 15 minutes
COOK TIME: 40 minutes

SERVINGS: 4
CARBS PER SERVING: 4 grams

When the work week is over, most of us are ready for a special "let's celebrate" dinner, but few of us have the energy (or the time) to make it. Here's a meal that will meet all your needs.

3 tablespoons olive oil
1 teaspoon chopped scallions
8 vegetable protein "steaklets" (found in many supermarket freezers), thawed per package directions
4 cloves garlic, crushed
2/3 cup heavy whipping cream

1/2 pound grated cheese (cheddar, American, Swiss, or Monterey Jack)
12 pitted green olives, drained and sliced
1 teaspoon Dijon mustard
1 teaspoon capers
Sour cream (optional)
Fresh parsley (optional)

Preheat the oven to 350°F.

Brush the inside of a deep ovenproof casserole dish with 1 table-spoon of the olive oil.

Heat the remaining 2 tablespoons of olive oil and the scallions in a large skillet over a medium flame. Sauté for 1 minute, stirring often, and then add the "steaklets."

Brown the "steaklets" (3 minutes per side), transfer to the bottom of the casserole dish, spread the crushed garlic on top of the "steaklets," and set aside. Retain the pan drippings in the skillet.

Add the cream to the skillet over a medium flame. Heat until the cream bubbles around the edges, then lower heat to medium-low before the cream comes to a full boil.

Add the cheese, a handful at a time, mixing well after each addition. Reduce heat even further and stir constantly, as this will be a very thick sauce.

Add the olive slices, mustard, and capers. Mix well and immediately pour the sauce over the "steaklets."

Bake, uncovered, for 30 minutes.

Remove the casserole from the oven and serve warm.

Garnish with a dollop of sour cream and fresh parsley.

Skillet Soufflé

PREP TIME: 13 minutes
COOK TIME: 20 minutes

SERVINGS: 4
CARBS PER SERVING: 2 grams

A super-satisfying breakfast, late-night snack or hearty meal anytime in between.

4 eggs, beaten
8 ounces cream cheese, quartered and softened
1/2 cup grated Parmesan or Romano cheese
2 tablespoons minced onion
2 tablespoons butter
1/4 cup chopped cilantro (optional)

1 package (10 ounces) frozen spinach, thawed and squeezed free of liquid
1/2 teaspoon ground white pepper
1/4 cup grated cheese (cheddar, American, Swiss, or Monterey Jack)
1 teaspoon paprika (hot or sweet)

In a small mixing bowl, combine the eggs, cream cheese, and Parmesan or Romano cheese. Mix well and set aside in the refrigerator.

Sauté the onion in the butter in a medium-size skillet over a medium flame, until the onion begins to brown (about 3 minutes).

Add the cilantro, spinach, and pepper. Mix well and cook until the entire mixture is warmed through, about 5 minutes.

Remove the skillet momentarily from the heat and, with a wooden spoon, spread the spinach mixture evenly across the bottom and up the sides of the skillet (to 1/2 inch from the top) to form a crust.

Remove the egg mixture from the refrigerator and stir once again. Keep the egg mixture in reach as the spinach skillet is returned to the fire.

Pour the egg mixture into the spinach crust into the skillet immediately.

Reduce heat to low, cover the skillet, and allow the soufflé to form and set, 8 to 10 minutes.

When the soufflé is formed (the egg mixture is cooked and no longer liquid in the middle), lift the cover on the skillet and sprinkle the cheese over the center. Garnish with the paprika.

(continued)

Remove the skillet from the heat, cover, and allow the cheese to melt.

Serve the soufflé warm, cutting in wedges using a pie cutter. Be careful to try to keep the spinach crust intact.

Mushroom Pâté

PREP TIME: 13 minutes
COOK TIME: 6 minutes

SERVINGS: 4
CARBS PER SERVING: 4 grams

At the Disneyland Hotel in Paris, the Inventions Restaurant welcomes you with a lunch and buffet that is purely French cuisine. One of our favorite dishes there inspired this pâté. We feel like our own honored guests when we sit back and enjoy its luxury.

2 tablespoons butter
2 tablespoons finely diced onion
2 cups finely diced fresh mushrooms
3 ounces cream cheese, quartered and softened
1 tablespoon capers

1/2 tablespoon marsala wine (optional)
1 tablespoon olive oil (more if needed)
Salt, pepper, and cayenne, as desired
Fresh parsley (optional)

Melt the butter in a medium-size saucepan and sauté the onion in the butter, stirring often, until it begins to brown (3 minutes). Add the mushrooms and continue to sauté, stirring often, until the mushrooms are soft and golden brown. Remove the pan from the heat. Using a slotted spoon, transfer the onions and mushrooms to a separate bowl, allowing the excess butter to drain off. Set them aside to cool.

In a food processor, combine 2 quarters of the cream cheese and the capers. Add one half of the mushroom mixture and the remainder of the cream cheese quarters, one at a time, processing well after each addition.

Add the marsala wine and process. Season with salt and pepper and cayenne. If needed, add olive oil to bring the mixture to a paste-like consistency.

Remove the mixture to a clean plate and, with wet hands, shape it into a pâté bar similar to the shape of an 8-ounce package of cream cheese. Garnish the bar with fresh parsley. Cover the pâté with an aluminum foil tent and refrigerate for 2 to 4 hours.

Serve with fresh cold celery or green bell pepper. This pâté is also perfect with our Tofu Crisps (page 103).

QUICK
FIXES

Instant Onion Dip

PREP TIME: 2 minutes

COOK TIME: 7 minutes

SERVINGS: 6 (¼ cup each)

CARBS PER SERVING: 3 grams

No need to use soup mixes or powdered blends. This 100 percent additive-free, sugar-free, easy-as-pie, and superbly delicious dip is ready when you are. We always keep a couple of small onions in the refrigerator, along with one or two small unopened containers of sour cream. When the urge hits, we have what we need right on hand.

1   teaspoon olive oil
½   cup finely chopped onion
1   cup sour cream

White pepper or hot sauce, as desired

Sparingly coat with the olive oil the bottom of a medium-size non-stick skillet. Add the chopped onion and heat over a medium-high flame until the onion caramelizes (turns deep brown), stirring constantly (about 7 minutes). Note: the onion will change from light brown to a dark caramel color quickly, so continue stirring and watch closely.

Remove the pan from the heat. Using a slotted spatula, remove the onion, draining and discarding all the oil. Transfer the caramelized onion to a medium-size bowl and allow it to cool completely.

Add the sour cream and stir well.

Add white pepper or hot sauce as desired.

Serve the dip cold with celery sticks, raw cauliflower, mushrooms, green pepper slices, or green beans, or as a topping for cooked meat, poultry, or seafood.

Fast Foo Young

PREP TIME: 6 minutes
COOK TIME: 6 minutes

SERVINGS: 4 (2 pancakes each)
CARBS PER SERVING: 2 grams

The perfect snack or quick lunch. We also love it for breakfast. Any cooked meat can be used in place of chicken, so it's a great way to use up leftovers as well.

8   eggs
1/4 pound string beans,
     trimmed
1   stalk celery
4   ounces cooked chicken
1/2 green bell pepper

3   medium-size mushrooms
1/4 small onion
2   teaspoons soy sauce
     Ground pepper and hot
     sauce, as desired
3   tablespoons olive oil

In a small bowl, beat the eggs well. Set aside.

Feed the string beans, celery, cooked chicken, green pepper, mushrooms, and onion into a food processor and process using the shredding blade. Add soy sauce and ground pepper and hot sauce. Use the pulse button and stop processing as soon as all large pieces are shredded.

Transfer the shredded ingredients to a large bowl and add the beaten egg. Mix well.

Divide the mixture into 8 portions (each person will get two portions).

Heat 1 teaspoon of the olive oil in a very large skillet, over a medium flame, until the oil is hot (but not smoking).

Carefully drop into the skillet by the spoonful one eighth of the egg mixture (oil may sputter). Smooth to form a flattened pancake and fry until the egg mixture is thoroughly cooked through and both sides are a deep golden brown. Repeat for all 8 portions.

If you're making a full recipe, use 2 skillets so that 2 servings can cook simultaneously and all of them can be ready at the same time.

Serve warm.

Savory Meal on a Stick

PREP TIME: 6 minutes

COOK TIME: none

SERVINGS: 4

CARBS PER SERVING: 1 to 3 grams
(depending on ingredients)

This dish is quick to make, and quicker to grab on the run. The ingredients are limited only by your imagination and your leftovers. The secret is to add just enough cream cheese to hold the ingredients together, and to vary the spices (and hot sauce) so the dish always tastes different.

1 cup total of any of the following, cooked very well, free of all shells or bones, and cut into 1-inch cubes:
    chicken
    turkey
    shrimp
    beef
    pork

1/4 cup total of any of the following:
    diced onions
    diced garlic
    diced scallions
    diced green bell pepper
    pitted green or black ripe olives, drained and sliced

Any of the following, as desired
    paprika (hot or sweet)
    hot sauce
    ground black or white pepper
    grated Parmesan or Romano cheese

4 ounces cream cheese

8 large celery stalks, cut into 4- to 5-inch sections

Combine the meat, vegetable, and spice ingredients of your choice in a food processor. Process to a chunky mixture.

Add the cream cheese and mix well with your hands to form a mixture that blends into a thick paste. Stuff the celery sections with the mixture.

Eat immediately, or keep refrigerated and eat within 2 to 3 hours of preparation.

Quick Kimchee

PREP TIME: 4 minutes

COOK TIME: 7 minutes

SERVINGS: 4

CARBS PER SERVING: 1 grams

The traditional preparation of this powerful condiment takes several days. This variation offers a fresh taste that's just as mighty but can be ready in only a fraction of the time.

3 cups finely shredded napa or green cabbage

1/2 cup olive oil

4 tablespoons butter

2 cloves garlic, minced (or 1 teaspoon garlic powder)

1/2 teaspoon crushed red pepper (or hot sauce, as desired)

Salt and ground black or white pepper, as desired

Place the cabbage in a large bowl and set aside.

Heat together the olive oil and butter in a large skillet over a moderate flame until they foam but are not brown (about 1 minute).

Reduce heat to low, add the garlic, and stir for 1 minute.

Add the pepper flakes (or hot sauce) and stir for 1 minute.

Remove the skillet from the heat and pour the warm butter mixture onto the cabbage. Mix very well to ensure an even distribution of the butter mixture.

Return the coated cabbage to the skillet and heat uncovered over a medium-high flame, stirring constantly, until the cabbage softens (about 4 minutes).

Remove the skillet from the heat and add salt and pepper as desired. Do not add salt until cooking is complete.

Serve as a condiment with meat, poultry, or seafood main dishes.

VARIATION

Add leftover cooked meat, poultry, or seafood, cut into 1-inch cubes, one minute before removing the finished dish from the heat. Continue to stir often.

Cheese Pop 'Ems

PREP TIME: 10 minutes

COOK TIME: none

SERVINGS: 4 (4 Pop 'Ems each)

CARBS PER SERVING: 1 gram

It might take you longer to read this recipe than to make it! These Cheese Pop 'Ems are quick, good, satisfying, and don't require a whole list of ingredients.

8 ounces cheddar cheese, cut into 1-inch chunks, softened

8 ounces cream cheese, quartered and softened

16 small pitted whole green or black ripe olives, drained

1/4 cup dried basil and/or paprika

In a large bowl combine the cheddar cheese and cream cheese. Mash the mixture with your hands to blend well. Divide the mixture into quarters, and each quarter into quarters, to form 16 equal portions. Set aside.

Pat dry the pitted olives with a paper towel. Take one portion of the cheese mixture and form a ball around an olive, leaving the olive as the center of the ball. Repeat until you've made 16 balls.

Sprinkle the basil and/or paprika sparsely on a baking sheet. Roll the cheese balls in the spice to coat.

(You may want to roll the balls with green olives in basil and those with black olives in paprika, so you know which balls hold each type of olive).

Refrigerate and serve cold.

Speedy Béarnaise

PREP TIME: 4 minutes

COOK TIME: 3 minutes

SERVINGS: 4 (3 tablespoons per serving)

CARBS PER SERVING: 2 grams

We used to be impressed with restaurants that served complicated sauces requiring long lists of ingredients and split-second timing. After years of experience we discovered the truth that you may already suspect: you can make a great sauce with a couple of ingredients and a few spare minutes. Best of all, a good sauce can turn any leftover into an instant meal. This recipe requires wine, so if that's not permitted on your diet, pass this one by.

4 scallions, finely chopped
3 tablespoons dry white wine
2 tablespoons white vinegar
1 teaspoon dried tarragon

Dash of salt and black pepper
2/3 cup sour cream

Combine the scallions, wine, vinegar, tarragon, and salt and pepper in a small saucepan over a medium flame. Bring to a soft boil, reduce the flame slightly, and cook for 1 minute.

Strain the mixture through a sieve or fine colander, discarding all solids and reserving the liquid.

Return the liquid to the saucepan and allow it to cool for 2 to 3 minutes.

Slowly stir in the sour cream, one dollop at a time, until all the sour cream has been incorporated into the liquid.

Heat over a low flame for 1 minute, until warm, stirring frequently. Do *not* bring to a boil.

Remove and serve immediately as a sauce for cooked meat, poultry, or seafood.

Swift Salmon and Dill Sauce

PREP TIME: 4 minutes

COOK TIME: 7 to 8 minutes

SERVINGS: 4

CARBS PER SERVING: 2 grams

This traditional dish already comes low-carb, but this is our easiest and favorite way to prepare it.

3 cups chicken stock (or our Classic Chicken Stock, page 66) or fish stock (or our Fundamental Fish Stock, page 185)

1/4 cup fresh dill stalks and leaves (do not chop)

1 teaspoon dill seed

1 teaspoon soy sauce

4 salmon steaks (4 to 6 ounces each), boneless

2 cups sour cream

In a large skillet combine the stock, fresh dill, dill seed, and soy sauce. Lay the salmon fillets in one layer across the bottom of the skillet, making certain the liquid covers the fish. If it doesn't, add enough water to barely cover the fillets. Remove the salmon before heating the liquid.

On a medium flame, heat the liquid to a boil.

Add the salmon and continue to heat. When the mixture again begins to boil, reduce heat to a gentle simmer and cook for 6 minutes, until the fish is completely cooked and flakes easily with a fork.

Remove the salmon to plates.

Strain the cooking stock through a coarse sieve or colander, allowing the seeds to pass through but not the dill. Set aside the dill and 1 tablespoon of retained cooking stock (without seeds).

In a small bowl, combine the sour cream, dill, and retained cooking stock. Mix well.

Top each salmon steak with 1 to 2 dollops of the sour cream mixture and serve immediately.

On-the-Run Tuna Salad Cups

PREP TIME: 6 minutes

COOK TIME: none

SERVINGS: 2

CARBS PER SERVING: 2 grams

When readers ask what they can have in place of sandwiches on a low-carb diet, we love to recommend our on-the-run cups. The variety is as limitless as your imagination, and you get the extra benefit of putting more vegetables into your diet without even trying. We frequently find ourselves doubling the recipe so we have some for now and some for later.

1 can (6½ ounces) tuna in water, drained

¼ cup peeled and diced cucumber

2 tablespoons diced onion

1 tablespoon mayonnaise

1 green bell pepper, cored, seeded, and cut in half

Paprika (hot or sweet), as desired

Grated Parmesan or Romano cheese, as desired

Mix the tuna, cucumber, onion, and mayonnaise in a medium-size bowl. Combine well to ensure even taste.

Stuff the tuna mixture in half a green pepper. Sprinkle with paprika or grated cheese as desired.

Keep refrigerated and enjoy ice cold while on the run.

VARIATIONS

Use any freshly cooked leftover poultry or meat, chopped in a small dice.

For a tasty, milder salad, add 1 hard-boiled egg, peeled. Mash the egg separately before adding.

Top with lettuce leaves or fresh sprigs of parsley.

Seafood Dijon Cobb Salad

PREP TIME: 15 minutes

COOK TIME: none

SERVINGS: 4

CARBS PER SERVING: 3 grams

We've found that the tangy taste of mustard and the smoky flavor of bacon bring out the best in shellfish and fowl. This dish is a summer classic at our house.

1 head romaine lettuce or spinach, washed, patted dry, and torn into bite-size pieces

2 tablespoons lemon juice

1½ tablespoons Dijon mustard

1 clove garlic, crushed
Salt and pepper, as desired

¼ cup olive oil

1 tablespoon chopped fresh parsley

4 ounces ready-to-eat canned king crab, drained

4 ounces ready-to-eat canned salad (tiny) shrimp, drained

4 ounces cheese of choice, chopped

4 eggs, hard-boiled, peeled, and quartered

4 slices bacon, cooked crisp and chopped

4 ounces cooked chicken or turkey, chopped

Place the greens in a large salad bowl. Set aside.

In a medium-size bowl, combine the lemon juice, mustard, garlic, and salt and pepper as desired.

Gradually add the olive oil, whisking constantly until the oil has been well incorporated. Add the parsley. Whisk well.

Pour the oil mixture onto the greens, one quarter of the mixture at a time, tossing well after each addition.

Top the salad with each of the remaining ingredients, laid in rows, side by side.

Serve ice cold.

Swift Cream of Asparagus Soup

PREP TIME: 4 minutes   SERVINGS: 2
COOK TIME: 8 minutes   CARBS PER SERVING: 3 grams

For when you want something warm and comforting and you want it now!

1 tablespoon butter	Salt, ground pepper, and
1/4 cup chopped onions	hot sauce, as desired
12 medium mushrooms, sliced	2 teaspoons arrowroot
1 can (8 1/4 ounces) asparagus	powder dissolved in
spears, chopped, without	4 teaspoons of water, for
liquid	thickening (optional)
2 cups heavy whipping cream	

Warm the butter in a medium-size saucepan over a medium flame, until bubbling (but not brown).

Turn the heat to low and add the onions. Sauté until the onions turn light golden brown (about 3 minutes), stirring often.

Add the mushrooms and continue to sauté and stir until softened and browning (about 3 minutes).

Add the chopped asparagus. Raise the heat to medium and bring the mixture to a soft boil.

Remove the pan from the heat immediately. Slowly add the cream, stirring constantly as you pour.

Add salt, ground pepper, and hot sauce as desired.

Transfer the mixture in batches to a food processor or blender and process until smooth, so that no chunks of vegetable remain.

If the soup has cooled, warm it back up slowly in a small saucepan on low heat. Warm only to the temperature appropriate for eating. Do *not* boil.

If desired, add the arrowroot and water mixture for thickening. Stir constantly to make certain the arrowroot mixture is distributed throughout.

Serve immediately, either alone or with our Tofu Crisps (page 103).

Soft and Speedy Brie

PREP TIME: 4 minutes
COOK TIME: 2 minutes

SERVINGS: 4 (2 rolls each)
CARBS PER SERVING: 1 gram

We put this dish together as an instant treat and now include it as an appetizer whenever we need something luscious.

8 spinach leaves, washed and patted dry
1/4 cup finely chopped celery
1 clove garlic, pressed
1 tablespoon dried basil

1 round (8 ounces) of brie cheese, cut into 8 equal wedges (you may remove the rind if you like, or leave it in place)
Hot sauce (optional)
Wooden toothpicks

Lay the spinach leaves out on a clean surface.

In a small bowl, mix the celery, garlic, and basil. Divide the celery mixture equally among all 8 spinach leaves, placing the mixture in the center of each leaf.

Place one wedge of brie at the end of a spinach leaf and fold over one side to cover the brie. Then roll the leaf, flattening the celery mixture as you go. Secure the leaf with a toothpick. Repeat the process for all 8 leaves.

Transfer all the spinach rolls to a steamer, placing each leaf seam side down (or place them on a rack in a covered skillet with 1 inch of water below the rack).

Steam the leaves on high (or at a rolling boil) for 2 minutes.

Remove the leaves from the heat and allow them to cool until they are comfortable to eat.

Remove the toothpicks and serve the spinach leaves warm. (Note: the brie remains hotter than the spinach leaf, so be careful of the hot cheese when taking your first bite.)

For extra flavor, dip the leaves in hot sauce.

Sausage Egg Cups

PREP TIME: 4
COOK TIME: 11 to 15 minutes

SERVINGS: 2 (2 cups each)
CARBS PER SERVING: 1 gram

If you don't have the time (or patience) to scramble eggs and cook up bacon for breakfast, here's an eye-opener that literally cooks itself. Wrap some large lettuce leaves around the finished cups and you can eat them on the go, though they're even better enjoyed with a relaxing cup of coffee or tea.

Nonstick cooking spray
4 patties sausage, fully cooked (or our Freedom Sausage, page 23, fully cooked)
1/4 cup grated cheese (cheddar, American, Swiss, or Monterey Jack)

4 eggs
2 teaspoons chopped celery, scallions, or fresh chives
Salt, pepper, and hot sauce, as desired

Preheat the oven to 350°F.

Spray 4 empty cups in a standard muffin tin with nonstick cooking spray and place a sausage patty in the bottom of each cup.

Sprinkle cheese on each sausage patty.

Break 1 egg into each cup.

Top with a sprinkle of celery, scallions, or chives, and season with salt, pepper, and hot sauce as desired.

Bake for 11 to 15 minutes, until the eggs are cooked throughout.

Place the muffin pan on a cake rack to cool for 2 minutes, then loosen the cups all around with a butter knife.

Slide each cup onto a plate or into a large lettuce leaf.

Serve warm, or cold as a grab-and-go breakfast treat.

Rapid Roquefort Cheese Sauce for Leftovers

PREP TIME: 3 minutes
COOK TIME: none

SERVINGS: 4 (¼ cup each)
CARBS PER SERVING: 1 gram

This luscious sauce turns last night's dinner into today's special treat.

1 stalk celery, diced (use one of the tender inner stalks)
1 clove garlic, peeled
1 tablespoon white vinegar
1 tablespoon dried basil
1 small scallion, minced

½ teaspoon paprika (hot or sweet)
¼ pound Roquefort cheese, cut in quarters
1 cup heavy cream

Place the celery, garlic, vinegar, basil, scallion, paprika, and Roquefort cheese into a blender or food processor. Add ¼ cup of the heavy cream. Purée or process.

Add the remainder of cream, ¼ cup at a time, puréeing or processing after each addition.

Enjoy cold or warm as a topping for cooked meats, poultry, seafood, or vegetables.

SMOOTH AND CREAMY

Deeply Good Creamed Mushrooms

PREP TIME: 3 minutes

COOK TIME: 7 minutes

SERVINGS: 4

CARBS PER SERVING: 3 grams

We were hoping to spice up our creamed mushroom recipe in preparation for a very special dinner we were planning. Our neighbor, Janice, was our guinea pig (in keeping with her standing request). When she tasted version #3, she smiled slowly and gave the dish its new name.

1/4 cup sour cream

1/4 cup mayonnaise

4 tablespoons grated Parmesan or Romano cheese

1 tablespoon basil
Salt and pepper, as desired

2 tablespoons butter

1 tablespoon olive oil

2 tablespoons diced onion

1 pound mushrooms, thinly sliced

2 tablespoons dry sherry (optional)
Additional grated Parmesan or Romano cheese, as desired
Fresh parsley or paprika (sweet or hot), as garnish

In a small bowl, place the sour cream, mayonnaise, Parmesan or Romano cheese, basil, and salt and pepper as desired. Mix well. Set aside.

Melt the butter and oil in a small skillet over a low-medium flame. Sauté the onion, stirring constantly, until it begins to brown around the edges.

Add the sliced mushrooms and sauté for 3 minutes, turning often.

Add the sherry, mix well, and cook for 1 minute.

Remove the skillet from the heat, allow to cool for 3 minutes, then slowly add the sour cream mixture to the mushrooms, blending well.

Return the skillet to a low flame and heat until the sour cream has warmed thoroughly (do not boil). Add additional grated cheese as desired.

Serve warm.

Garnish with fresh parsley or sprinkle with paprika.

Left Bank Boursin

PREP TIME: 4 minutes
COOK TIME: none

SERVINGS: 6 (2 ounces each)
CARBS PER SERVING: 1 gram

We never considered making Boursin (French herbed cheese) at home; somehow we always assumed it would be an involved process, like the making of cheese itself. A friend brought us a recipe from a little café in Paris where the only dish on the menu was baked potatoes heaped with Boursin. We adapted it slightly, and now we can't imagine ever buying Boursin in the store again.

1 stick butter, quartered and softened
8 ounces cream cheese, quartered and softened
1 1/2 teaspoons minced fresh parsley (or 1/2 teaspoon parsley flakes)

1/2 teaspoon ground white pepper
1/2 teaspoon garlic powder
1/2 teaspoon dried marjoram

Cream the butter in a medium-size bowl, adding one chunk at a time. Add the cream cheese, one chunk at a time, thoroughly creaming the two together.

Add the spices and mix well.

Cover the bowl and refrigerate overnight.

Serve as a vegetable dip, as stuffing for celery, or as a spread on meats, fish, poultry, or cooked vegetables.

VARIATIONS

As you are adding the herbs, add 1 tablespoon grated Parmesan or Romano cheese or 1/2 teaspoon prepared horseradish.

Great on low-carb Mashed "Potatoes" (page 210).

Olive Cheese Spread

PREP TIME: 5 minutes

COOK TIME: none

SERVINGS: 4 (¼ cup each)

CARBS PER SERVING: 1 gram

Going to New York City is just an excuse to visit Avra and indulge in the best of fine Greek cuisine. One dish we enjoyed there inspired us to come up with this recipe, although we still make excuses to return to New York so we can enjoy the real thing.

3 ounces cream cheese,
   quartered and softened
1 can (3¼ ounces) small
   pitted black ripe or green
   olives, sliced, liquid retained

2 teaspoons grated onion
½ cup mayonnaise
½ cup grated cheddar cheese
   or jalapeño American
   cheese

In a medium-size bowl (or electric mixing bowl), blend the cream cheese quarters until soft.

Add the olive slices and 1 tablespoon of liquid from the olives. Blend well.

Add the remaining ingredients, mixing well after each addition.

Serve cold as stuffing for celery, as a filling for lettuce pockets, or as a dip for our Tofu Crisps (page 103).

Must-Taste Salmon Mousse

PREP TIME: 5 minutes
COOK TIME: none

SERVINGS: 2 (1/2 cup each)
CARBS PER SERVING: 1 gram

This sophisticated mousse takes on the satisfying flavor of good ol' snack food when served with our Crisp and Crackly Cheese Crackers (page 104) or our Tofu Crisps (page 103). Once you've made this dish, you'll find yourself keeping canned salmon on the shelf at all times . . . just in case. This one is special and quick.

1 teaspoon fresh dill
2 tablespoons fresh parsley
2 tablespoons chopped scallions
1 can (7.5 ounces) red salmon, drained, bones and skin removed

1 tablespoon lemon juice
1 tablespoon mayonnaise
1/2 tablespoon sour cream
1/2 tablespoon Dijon mustard
    Salt and ground pepper, as desired

Place all the ingredients in a blender or food processor and purée or process just until the mixture becomes smooth and creamy.

Transfer to a small bowl, cover, and refrigerate for several hours or overnight.

Serve ice cold.

Cheesy Creamed Spinach

PREP TIME: 4 minutes

COOK TIME: 7 to 10 minutes

SERVINGS: 4

CARBS PER SERVING: 1 gram

Rachael: *Richard and I had a disagreement. I knew I was wrong, but I wasn't going to admit it. I made this dish, one of his favorites, and he understood. Even better, he gave me a hug and never mentioned it again.*

2 tablespoons butter
2 cloves garlic, crushed
1 package (10 ounces) frozen chopped spinach, thawed and squeezed free of liquid

1/2 cup grated American or cheddar cheese
2 tablespoons heavy whipping cream
Salt, ground pepper, and hot sauce, as desired

In a large skillet over a low-medium flame heat the butter to bubbling but not brown. Reduce heat to low.

Add the garlic, stirring well, and sauté for 1 minute.

Raise heat to medium. Add the spinach, a handful at a time, stirring well after each addition to distribute the garlic evenly and heat well (4 to 6 minutes).

When the spinach is hot all the way through, gradually add the cheese, about 2 tablespoons at a time, mixing constantly while you continue to heat the mixture (about 2 more minutes). The spinach will become creamy and thick with cheese.

Add the cream, 1/2 tablespoon at a time, continuing to heat and stir until the mixture is creamy and smooth (about 30 seconds).

Add salt, pepper, and hot sauce as desired.

Serve warm.

Velvety Almond Whip

PREP TIME: 5 minutes
COOK TIME: none

SERVINGS: 2
CARBS PER SERVING: 2 grams

We like this simple smoothie ice cold. When you're in the mood for something silky but you want a low-carb treat without a sugar substitute, you can whip this one up in minutes.

1   cup sour cream
3   ounces cream cheese,
      quartered
1/4 teaspoon almond extract

1/4 teaspoon vanilla
Heavy whipping cream as needed
Dash of cinnamon

Place the sour cream in an electric mixing bowl. Add the cream cheese quarters, one at a time, mixing at high speed after each addition. Continue to blend at high speed until fluffy.

Add the almond extract and vanilla and mix.

Whip at high speed, adding the heavy whipping cream, 1 tablespoon at a time, until a soft cloudlike texture is reached.

Serve in tall iced tea glasses with spoons. Garnish with a sprinkle of cinnamon.

Cream of Asparagus Soufflé

PREP TIME: 7 minutes

COOK TIME: 45 to 50 minutes

SERVINGS: 4

CARBS PER SERVING: 3 grams

The secret to the silkiness of this dish is in the timing. Start the baking process so that you'll be ready to enjoy the soufflé as soon as it has cooled enough to eat.

Nonstick cooking spray

1 pound asparagus, trimmed of tough ends and cut into 2-inch lengths

2 tablespoons butter, at room temperature

4 eggs

1/2 cup grated Parmesan or Romano cheese

1 tablespoon capers

1/2 teaspoon salt

1/4 teaspoon ground black pepper

Hot sauce or chili oil, as desired

1 cup sour cream

1 teaspoon chopped fresh dill

Preheat the oven to 350°F.

Spray a medium-size ovenproof baking dish with nonstick cooking spray. Set aside.

Heat 1 1/2 inches of water to boiling in a medium-size saucepan over a medium flame. Add the asparagus and boil for 5 minutes. Drain and discard the cooking liquid.

Transfer the asparagus to a blender or food processor and purée or process until fully blended, with no chunks visible. Add the butter and blend again.

Add the eggs, Parmesan or Romano, capers, salt, pepper, and hot sauce or chili oil as desired, and process until the mixture is thick and smooth.

With a spatula, transfer the asparagus mixture to the prepared baking dish.

Bake for 40 to 45 minutes, until the center is no longer liquid and is set.

Serve warm. Top each serving with a dollop of sour cream and a sprinkling of dill.

Nova Scotia Scallops

PREP TIME: 5 minutes

COOK TIME: 13 minutes

SERVINGS: 2

CARBS PER SERVING: 2 grams

Rachael: *We arrived at the hotel in Halifax at exactly 10 P.M., the same time the restaurant closed. Room service didn't look promising—lots of gourmet-style food when I wanted good old-fashioned satisfaction. Finally, I noticed the dish that inspired this recipe, which was just what the doctor ordered: lots of protein and great taste.*

2 tablespoons butter
1 tablespoon olive oil
2 cloves garlic, pressed
2 tablespoons capers
1/2 cup heavy whipping cream

3/4 pound raw sea scallops,
washed and patted dry
1 teaspoon soy sauce
Paprika (hot or sweet), as
desired and for garnish

Over low heat, in a medium-size saucepan (not a skillet), warm the butter until it is foamy but not brown (1 minute).

Add the olive oil and garlic. Mix and heat until the olive oil is hot (but not smoking) and the garlic is fragrant (about 2 minutes).

Add the capers and stir for 1 minute.

Add the cream and raise the heat to medium. Stir the mixture to prevent sticking and continue to heat it until the cream reaches a full boil (about 3 minutes).

Add the scallops one at a time, stirring constantly.

Cook for 4 minutes after the last scallop has been added.

Season with the soy sauce and paprika as desired, and cook 2 minutes longer.

Using a slotted spoon, transfer the scallops to a shallow serving bowl. Discard the remaining cream.

Sprinkle the scallops with more paprika as a garnish and serve warm.

Quick Creamy Blue Cheese Dip

PREP TIME: 4 minutes

COOK TIME: none

SERVINGS: 8 (2 tablespoons each)

CARBS PER SERVING: 1 gram

It seems we've been making and enjoying this recipe for decades. It's a standard at our house, served almost every day, with fresh vegetables or salad before our main meal. Still, we never get tired of it.

1 cup creamy cottage cheese

2 ounces blue cheese, crumbled

1 teaspoon dried basil (or 1 tablespoon chopped fresh basil)

1/4 teaspoon ground black pepper

1 clove garlic, pressed

1/2 cup sour cream

Place the cottage cheese, blue cheese, basil, pepper, and garlic in a food processor, blender, or mixer, and blend at high speed until the mixture is smooth and creamy.

Fold in the sour cream, mixing well.

Transfer the mixture to a small bowl, cover, and refrigerate for 2 hours.

Serve cold with crudités (finger salad of raw green beans, wax beans, snap beans, green pepper slices, cauliflower florets, mushroom caps, and cucumber slices) or pour over a crisp green salad.

Also excellent as a dip for cold or hot meat, poultry, and seafood.

Sweet and Savory Pork Chops

PREP TIME: 12 minutes

COOK TIME: 25 minutes

SERVINGS: 4

CARBS PER SERVING: 2 grams

Richard: I love pork chops, but Rachael doesn't like meat that has even a hint of a gamy taste. We found the perfect way to satisfy us both. Soaking the chops in milk before cooking them gets rid of any gamy flavor that might be lurking, and this recipe provides us with a taste that's almost impossible to resist.

4 pork chops, loin, 1/2 inch thick

1 quart milk

4 tablespoons olive oil

1/4 cup chopped onion

4 slices bacon, cooked crisp and crumbled

1 teaspoon dried basil (or 1 tablespoon fresh basil)

1/2 cup heavy whipping cream

Salt and pepper, as desired

Parsley, as garnish

Three to five hours prior to preparing this dish, place the pork chops in a shallow bowl and cover completely with milk. Cover the bowl and place it in the refrigerator. Periodically turn the chops to ensure that all sides are exposed to the milk. (Wash hands and utensils well after any exposure to raw or undercooked pork.)

Remove the pork from the refrigerator and drain and discard all the milk. Wash the pork chops under running water and return them to the rinsed bowl.

Heat the olive oil in a large skillet over medium heat until hot (but not smoking). Add the onion and cook, stirring often, until golden brown. Add the bacon and basil and stir for 1 minute, scraping and stirring any brown bits from the pan.

Add the pork chops. Brown and cook well, about 10 minutes on each side, until the meat is thoroughly cooked and not pink at all.

Remove the pork chops to a clean, dry plate and cover them to retain their heat.

Add the cream to the skillet, still on medium heat, and stir to dislodge brown bits and juices. Mix well with the cream.

Add salt and pepper, as desired.

(continued)

Reduce the heat to low-medium and continue to cook the liquid for 2 minutes.

Pour the liquid over the chops. Top with parsley garnish. Cover to enhance the absorption of the warm, creamy liquid.

Allow the chops to remain covered for 3 minutes, then serve warm.

Silken Cream of Turkey Soup

PREP TIME: 2 minutes
COOK TIME: 30 minutes

SERVINGS: 2 (1 cup each)
CARBS PER SERVING: 4 grams

Thanksgiving leftovers can be transformed into a thick soup that is almost better than the freshly roasted turkey.

3 tablespoons butter
2 cloves garlic, minced
1/4 cup chopped onion
1 cup chicken stock (or our Classic Chicken Stock, page 66)
3 cups cooked turkey (or chicken) meat, skin and bones removed, shredded into strings or cut into 1/2-inch cubes
1 tablespoon dried basil

1 teaspoon dried rosemary
Salt, pepper, and hot sauce, as desired
4 slices bacon, cooked crisp (optional)
1 cup diced celery
2 teaspoons arrowroot powder dissolved in 4 teaspoons of water, for thickening (optional)
1 cup heavy whipping cream

Melt the butter in a medium-size saucepan over low-medium heat, to foaming but not brown. Add the garlic and onion. Cook until the garlic is fragrant and the onion turns translucent (3 to 5 minutes).

Add the stock, turkey, basil, rosemary, salt, pepper, and hot sauce as desired, and bacon, stirring well after each addition. Continue to cook at a slow simmer for 20 minutes.

Reduce the heat to low. Add the celery. Cover and cook until the celery is tender but not mushy (about 5 minutes).

Remove the pan from the heat. If desired, add the arrowroot mixture for thickening. Stir constantly to make certain the arrowroot mixture is distributed throughout.

Add the cream, stir gently, and serve warm.

VARIATIONS

Don't be afraid to add unusual low-carb vegetables such as frozen spinach (thawed and squeezed dry), asparagus, green beans (trimmed and added at the same time as the celery), or the green part of scallions (also nice as a garnish).

Or, add 1/2 cup of diced cooked cauliflower, green beans, or spinach along with the turkey.

Smooth and Cheesy Crabmeat Casserole

PREP TIME: 15 minutes	SERVINGS: 4
COOK TIME: 10 minutes	CARBS PER SERVING: 3 grams

Rachael: Our biggest disagreement over this sauce is which cheese to use in the recipe. Richard loves Swiss; I prefer American. He usually gives in . . . then I feel guilty. No problem. Once we take our first bite, we're in heaven.

Nonstick cooking spray
3 tablespoons butter
2 scallions, green part only, diced
1 clove garlic, minced
1/2 cup minced green bell pepper
1/2 cup minced celery
1 teaspoon paprika (hot or sweet)
1 pound cooked crabmeat, cartilage and shell completely removed
6 tablespoons heavy whipping cream
1 package (10 ounces) frozen spinach, thawed and squeezed free of liquid

Cheese Sauce

3 teaspoons butter
1 cup light whipping cream
Salt, pepper, and cayenne as desired
3/4 cup grated cheese (cheddar, American, Swiss, or Monterey Jack)

Preheat the oven to 250°F.

Spray a medium-size ovenproof casserole dish with nonstick cooking spray. Put aside.

In a medium-size skillet over a medium flame, melt the butter and sauté the scallions, garlic, green pepper, celery, and paprika, for 5 to 7 minutes (until the scallions, green pepper, and celery soften and the garlic becomes fragrant). Do not allow the butter to burn.

Add the crabmeat, whipping cream, and spinach, stirring well to distribute the butter mixture.

Transfer the entire mixture to the casserole dish. Place the casserole dish, covered, into the oven to keep warm.

(continued)

To make the Cheese Sauce, melt the butter in a small saucepan over a low flame.

Raise the heat to medium. Add the whipping cream and salt, pepper, and cayenne as desired and heat, stirring often, until bubbles form around the edges of the liquid. Do not allow the cream to stick to the bottom of the pan or to come to a boil.

Turn the heat to low and add the cheese, one third at a time, stirring constantly.

As soon as the cheese has melted into the cream, remove the pan from the heat, continuing to stir.

Remove the crabmeat casserole from the oven and pour the sauce over the crabmeat.

Serve immediately.

Quick Spinach Alfredo Pockets

PREP TIME: 13 minutes
COOK TIME: 15 minutes

SERVINGS: 4
CARBS PER SERVING: 1 gram

We try to schedule time to eat in peace and quiet, but sometimes life refuses to cooperate and it's eat on the run or not at all. For the busiest times in our lives, this recipe has proven to be a lifesaver.

1 teaspoon salt
4 green cabbage leaves
3 tablespoons butter
3 cloves garlic, crushed
1/3 cup heavy whipping cream

1/2 package (10 ounces) frozen spinach, thawed and squeezed free of liquid
1 can (6 ounces) mushroom slices, drained well
1/4 cup grated Parmesan or Romano cheese

Fill a large pot with 3 quarts of water and 1 teaspoon salt. Place, covered, over a high flame.

When the water comes to a boil, drop in the large cabbage leaves, stir to ensure they are covered, and replace the cover on the pot.

Boil the leaves for 5 minutes or until they are softened but still retain a hint of crispness.

Drain the cabbage leaves with a colander and immediately run cold water over them to stop the cooking process. Dry the leaves with a paper towel and arrange them flat on a clean, dry surface.

Melt the butter in a medium-size skillet over a medium flame and sauté the garlic in it for 3 minutes, stirring often.

Add the cream and continue to heat, stirring occasionally, until bubbles appear around the edges of the skillet (about 3 minutes).

Add the spinach, 1 handful at a time, stirring well after each addition. Continue to heat and stir (to prevent burning) until the spinach mixture is hot but not boiling (about 4 minutes).

Remove the skillet from the heat and add the mushrooms and cheese. Stir very well.

Spoon an equal portion of the spinach mixture into the center of each wilted cabbage leaf.

Fold into pockets and serve warm.

Vanilla Clouds

PREP TIME: 3 minutes
COOK TIME: 8 minutes

SERVINGS: 4
CARBS PER SERVING: 0 grams

A quick-fix no-carb treat that you can make in minutes. Perfect when you're craving a legal dessert—with no sugar substitute!

2 egg whites
1/2 teaspoon vanilla extract

1/2 cup olive oil

Allow the egg whites to come to room temperature. Transfer them to the bowl of an electric mixer. To maximize egg white peaks, make certain the bowl is completely dry.

Beat the egg whites at medium speed until stiff peaks form. Do not overbeat to dryness.

Fold in the vanilla extract, cutting into the peaks with a spatula, so that the peaks remain intact.

In a medium-size skillet over a medium flame, heat the olive oil until hot (but not smoking).

Drop dollops of the egg white mixture into the hot oil. Do not disturb them until the edges brown.

Once the dollops are browned well on one side (about 5 minutes), turn them gently, using a spatula and a spoon.

Cook on the other side until golden brown (another 3 minutes). When all surfaces are well browned, transfer the "clouds" to a paper-towel-lined plate to drain for 1 to 2 minutes. Do not pat with paper towel. Serve as soon as the "clouds" cool.

SPICY HOT SATISFACTION

Homemade Hot Sauce

PREP TIME: 5 minutes

COOK TIME: 6 to 7 minutes

SERVINGS: yields 1 cup (serving size ⅛ teaspoon)

CARBS PER SERVING: 0 grams

A good basic seasoning we use whenever hot sauce is called for.

¼ pound (2 to 3) fresh red chili peppers*, seeded and finely chopped	½ cup white vinegar ½ teaspoon salt

In a small nonreactive saucepan (ideally stainless steel; do not use an aluminum or nonstick pan) over a medium flame, heat the chopped peppers and vinegar. Stir, add salt, and heat the mixture.

Reduce the heat to low and simmer (at a soft boil) for 5 to 6 minutes, stirring occasionally. Remove the pan from the heat and allow the mixture to cool.

Transfer the mixture to a blender or food processor. Purée until it is smooth, adding more vinegar if necessary to achieve the right consistency.

Strain the mixture through a fine sieve. Transfer it to a screw-top glass bottle and store it in the refrigerator.

*NOTE: When handling chili peppers, it's always a good idea to wear rubber or latex gloves. The pepper can burn and irritate your hands even if you are not aware of any tiny cuts or abrasions that may exist. Be certain not to touch your face or eyes or any other area that may be vulnerable to damage or irritation. Immediately wash knife, cutting surfaces, and gloves when finished.

New Orleans Smoke and Fire

PREP TIME: 7 minutes
COOK TIME: 4 minutes

SERVINGS: yields 1 cup (serving size ⅛ teaspoon)
CARBS PER SERVING: 0 grams

The slightly burned flavor infused with garlic gives this sauce a special smoky taste.

1 tablespoon olive oil	1 clove garlic, pressed
¼ pound (2 to 3) fresh green chili peppers*, seeded and split in half	½ cup white vinegar
	½ teaspoon salt

Preheat the broiler.

Pour the olive oil into a shallow bowl.

Wearing rubber or latex gloves, dip each strip of green chili pepper into the olive oil and then place it on a foil-lined baking sheet.

Broil the pepper strips for 4 minutes or until the skins begin to brown all over (but are not burned).

After roasting, immediately place the peppers in a paper bag, seal, and allow them to steam for 15 minutes. Open the paper bag and allow the pepper strips to cool.

When the peppers are cool enough to handle (still wearing gloves), peel away the pepper skins and discard them.

Transfer the peppers and garlic to a blender or food processor. While blending or processing, add the vinegar in a slow, steady stream. Add the salt.

Continue processing until the mixture is completely blended.

Pour the sauce into a screw-top bottle and keep refrigerated.

*NOTE: When handling chili peppers, it's always a good idea to wear rubber or latex gloves. The pepper can burn and irritate your hands even if you are not aware of any tiny cuts or abrasions that may exist. Be certain not to touch your face or eyes or any other area that may be vulnerable to damage or irritation. Immediately wash knife, cutting surfaces, and gloves when finished.

Hawaiian Hot-Hot Sauce

PREP TIME: 7 minutes

COOK TIME: 2 minutes

SERVINGS: yields 1 cup (serving size 1/8 teaspoon)

CARBS PER SERVING: 0 grams

Scuba diving on an island with only a few dozen permanent inhabitants and one lunch counter attached to the airport, we told ourselves that we were there for the sport and not the food, which was wholesome but ordinary. The hot sauce served there, however, made it all worthwhile. Here's our version.

1/4 pound (2 to 3) fresh green or red chili peppers*, seeded	1/2 tablespoon Dijon mustard
1 clove garlic, pressed	1/4 teaspoon dried allspice
2 tablespoons diced tomato (optional)	1/4 teaspoon salt
	1/2 cup lime juice

To blanch the peppers, place a medium-size saucepan half-filled with water over a medium flame. Bring the water to a boil. Wearing latex or rubber gloves, drop the peppers into the boiling water for 2 minutes exactly. Drain the peppers in a colander and immediately flood with cold water. Continue running cold water over the peppers until they are cool. Drain all water.

Still wearing gloves, remove the peppers and apply pressure so that skins peel off. Discard the skins.

Transfer the peppers, along with the garlic, tomato, mustard, allspice, and salt, to a blender or food processor. While blending or processing, add the lime juice in a slow, steady stream.

Continue processing until the mixture is completely blended. Add additional lime juice as needed for desired consistency.

Pour the sauce into a screw-top jar and refrigerate.

*NOTE: When handling chili peppers, it's always a good idea to wear rubber or latex gloves. The pepper can burn and irritate your hands even if you are not aware of any tiny cuts or abrasions that may exist. Be certain not to touch your face or eyes or any other area that may be vulnerable to damage or irritation. Immediately wash knife, cutting surfaces, and gloves when finished.

Chimichurri Veal

PREP TIME: 7 minutes

COOK TIME: 25 to 60 minutes

SERVINGS: 4

CARBS PER SERVING: 1 gram

We had no idea what Argentinian food was like until friends threw us a small anniversary party at a restaurant famous for its authentic cuisine. After one taste, we knew we had to find a way to recreate the Argentinian flavors that are known as chimichurri.

1/2 cup olive oil	1 tablespoon fresh red or green chili peppers*, finely minced (or 1 teaspoon cayenne)
1/4 cup lemon juice	
1/4 cup finely diced onion	
2 cloves garlic, minced	
3 scallions, chopped	1 teaspoon salt
1/3 cup minced fresh parsley	4 veal cutlets (4 ounces), boneless
1 teaspoon dried oregano	

Combine all the ingredients except the cutlets in a large, shallow bowl.

Add the cutlets, being certain that the marinade entirely covers the meat.

Refrigerate, covered, for at least 2 hours.

Grill the marinated cutlets over a medium flame, basting with the marinade and turning the meat frequently until it is thoroughly cooked.

As an alternative, bake the cutlets in the oven at 350°F for 50 minutes, turning and basting the meat once after 15 minutes. Continue baking until the meat is fully cooked. Reset the oven to broil and finish by broiling for an additional 5 minutes on each side.

*NOTE: When handling chili peppers, it's always a good idea to wear rubber or latex gloves. The pepper can burn and irritate your hands even if you are not aware of any tiny cuts or abrasions that may exist. Be certain not to touch your face or eyes or any other area that may be vulnerable to damage or irritation. Immediately wash knife, cutting surfaces, and gloves when finished.

Hot and Puffy Lamb Chops

PREP TIME: 5 minutes
COOK TIME: 1 hour

SERVINGS: 4
CARBS PER SERVING: 1 gram

The Storyteller's Café at Disney's Grand Californian Hotel has become our shrine for good food: breakfast, lunch, and dinner. We used to order an incredible pork chop dish there that inspired this recipe. We were not happy when the restaurant came out with an entirely new menu, until we discovered that their newest creations are even better than our old favorites.

1/2 teaspoon crushed red pepper
1 teaspoon mayonnaise
4 tablespoons olive oil
4 pork chops, loin, about 3/4 inch thick
2 tablespoons soy sauce

1 tablespoon dried tarragon
1 teaspoon garlic powder
1 teaspoon paprika (hot or sweet)
2 tablespoons Dijon mustard
Salt and ground pepper, as desired

In a small bowl, combine the crushed red pepper and mayonnaise. Put the mixture aside in the refrigerator.

Preheat the oven to 350°F.

Spread 1 tablespoon of the olive oil in a broiler pan. Lay the pork chops in the pan, in a single layer, and drizzle them with the remaining olive oil, followed by the soy sauce.

Remove the bowl containing the mayonnaise mixture from the refrigerator and add the tarragon, garlic powder, paprika, mustard, and salt and pepper as desired. Mix well.

Divide the mayonnaise mixture among all four chops and spread it generously on top.

Bake the chops for 55 minutes.

Reset the oven temperature to broil and move the pan to the broiler. Watch carefully to avoid burning and broil the top of the chops until they rise to form a puffy crust (2 to 5 minutes).

Remove the pan from the oven, transfer the chops to a serving platter, and serve warm.

Mexican Pizza

PREP TIME: 10 minutes
COOK TIME: 20 to 25 minutes

SERVINGS: 4
CARBS PER SERVING: 1 to 4 grams
(depending on toppings)

The secret to this special recipe lies in the flavor the cayenne adds. The fiery taste works well to perk up the low-carb vegetables and other toppings.

3/4 pound ground hamburger
3 tablespoons grated
    Parmesan or Romano
    cheese
3 cloves garlic, minced
1 teaspoon dried oregano

1 tablespoon dried basil
1/2 teaspoon cayenne (or as
    desired to add lots of
    spice and flavor)
3/4 cup grated mozzarella

Low-Carb Toppings:

Mushrooms, caps or sliced
(raw, canned, or sautéed)
Green bell pepper, sliced thin
Pitted sliced black ripe
olives, drained

Grated Parmesan or
Romano cheese
Diced fresh tomato (no
more than 2 tablespoons)

Preheat the oven to broil.

In a medium-size mixing bowl, using your hands, thoroughly combine the hamburger, grated cheese, garlic, oregano, basil, and cayenne.

Press the meat mixture into a 9-inch pie pan (preferably glass) so that the sides and bottom are evenly covered.

Place the pan under the broiler for 15 minutes. Make sure the meat crust browns and dries out but does not burn. Remove the pan from the oven and carefully pour off any liquid or grease that might have been released by cooking.

Reduce oven temperature to 350°F, for baking.

To the meat crust add low-carb toppings, as desired.

Finish with a generous layer of grated mozzarella.

Return to the oven and bake for 6 to 8 minutes, until top cheese layer has melted well.

Remove and serve warm, cut in wedges.

Blazing Ribs

PREP TIME: 7 minutes
COOK TIME: 2 hours

SERVINGS: 4
CARBS PER SERVING: 1 gram

Warming the crushed red pepper with three different oils and using a variety of herbs infuses spicy flavor that seeps into these ribs as they cook. We have certain friends who request a repeat of this dish whenever they're invited to our house for dinner.

2 tablespoons sesame oil
2 tablespoons peanut oil
1/4 cup olive oil
1 tablespoon soy sauce
1 teaspoon lemon juice
3 cloves garlic, minced
1/4 teaspoon ground coriander

1/4 teaspoon ground turmeric
1/4 teaspoon dried basil
1/4 teaspoon dried marjoram
1 teaspoon crushed red pepper
3 1/2 pounds country ribs (beef or pork)

In a small saucepan over low heat, warm all the oils, the soy sauce, lemon juice, garlic, coriander, turmeric, basil, marjoram, and crushed red pepper for 2 minutes only.

Remove the pan from the heat and set it aside to cool.

Transfer the ribs to a larger, deep container. Pour (and rub) the cooled oil mixture on all rib surfaces. (Throughout the preparation, wash your hands and all dishes and utensils after contact with raw or undercooked pork.)

Allow the ribs to marinate for at least 2 hours, basting with marinade drippings.

Preheat the oven to 375°F.

Place the ribs on a rack over a roasting pan and pour the marinade over them.

Bake for 2 hours, until the meat is thoroughly cooked and pulls easily away from the bone.

Flaming Shrimp Portobello

PREP TIME: 7 minutes
COOK TIME: 1 to 2 minutes

SERVINGS: 2 to 4
CARBS PER SERVING: 1 to 2 grams

We visited Page, Arizona, in order to see the magnificent Antelope Slot Canyon. What we didn't expect to find, however, was a five-star restaurant among the storefronts in town. The restaurant's signature appetizer inspired us to go home and create our own spicy seafood version.

2 portobello mushrooms
1 tablespoon sesame oil
3 teaspoons butter, softened
3 ounces cream cheese, cut into quarters and softened
1 teaspoon hot sauce (or 3 drops chili oil), or as desired
1/4 teaspoon black pepper

1 teaspoon white prepared horseradish
1 teaspoon pressed garlic
1 1/2 pounds shrimp, cooked, shelled, and deveined, cut into 1-inch chunks
2 teaspoons olive oil
Cayenne or paprika (hot or sweet) as desired

Preheat the oven to broil.

Coat the curved caps of the portobello mushrooms with sesame oil. Place inverted on a flat baking sheet. Put aside.

Into a food processor or blender, put the butter, cream cheese, hot sauce, pepper, horseradish, garlic, shrimp, and olive oil. Process or blend until the mixture becomes a paste with lumps of shrimp. (If necessary, add an additional teaspoon of olive oil.)

Mound the shrimp mixture in the mushroom cups. Sprinkle with cayenne or paprika, as desired.

Place the mushrooms under the broiler for 1 to 2 minutes to warm, being careful not to burn the edges.

Blazing Broccoli Rabe and Shrimp

PREP TIME: 2 minutes
COOK TIME: 10 minutes

SERVINGS: 4
CARBS PER SERVING: 4 grams

Broccoli rabe is a leafy mustard green that echoes the tang that runs in this family of plants. Also called rapini, broccoli raab, and sprouting broccoli, this vegetable was prized as a delicacy by Roman centurions more than two thousand years ago. Though exotic and timeless, it can probably be found in your local supermarket or produce store.

1 pound broccoli rabe, roughly chopped
2 teaspoons salt
2 large garlic cloves, pressed
16 medium shrimp, raw, shelled and deveined

2 tablespoons olive oil
Hot sauce or chili oil, as desired

Pour 3 quarts of water into a large saucepan and bring to a boil over a medium-high flame.

Add the broccoli rabe and salt and cook until the greens are wilted and tender (about 3 minutes).

Remove the pan from the heat, drain the broccoli rabe in a colander, and run cold water over the greens to immediately stop the cooking process. Set the colander aside to continue to drain.

Stir-fry the garlic and shrimp in the olive oil in a medium-size skillet over a medium-high flame.

When the shrimp is completely cooked (white and opaque) (about 6 minutes), add the broccoli rabe, stirring to combine with the garlic, oil, and shrimp, and until the greens are heated through (about 1 minute).

Season with a hot sauce or chili oil of your choice as desired (not crushed red peppers), to make a pleasurably fiery dish.

Longboat Key Lime Steak

PREP TIME: 12 minutes
COOK TIME: 13 minutes

SERVINGS: 4
CARBS PER SERVING: 2 grams

Brunch at the Colony Beach and Tennis Resort in Sarasota, Florida, involves choosing from an amazing buffet that includes at least three dozen perfectly prepared dishes. We adapted this dish from one of our favorites so we didn't have to wait until our next visit to enjoy it.

1 pound steak, sirloin or strip, pounded thin
Nonstick cooking spray (or 2 tablespoons olive oil)
4 dashes hot sauce (or 8 drops of chili oil), as desired
1/4 cup minced scallions
1/2 cup sliced mushrooms
1 cup crushed pork rinds (optional)

2 tablespoons dried basil (or 1/4 cup chopped fresh basil)
1/4 teaspoon ground ginger
2 cloves garlic, peeled and halved
2 tablespoons Key lime juice (or lime juice)
Wooden toothpicks
2 tablespoons olive oil
2 tablespoons soy sauce

Cut the steak into 4 pieces of equal size.

Spray a baking sheet with nonstick cooking spray. Lay each section of steak flat on the baking sheet and spread 1 to 2 dashes of hot sauce on top of each steak.

Place in the refrigerator.

Preheat the broiler.

Place the scallions, mushrooms, pork rinds, basil, ginger, and garlic in a large Ziploc bag. Close well and gently apply pressure with a rolling pin or the roll of a fist until the pork rinds are pulverized to breadcrumb size and the scallions and spices are well mixed. Set aside.

Remove the steaks from the refrigerator. Drizzle the lime juice equally on all 4 steaks.

Divide the pork rind mixture equally among the steaks, placing a mound of mixture 1/2 inch in from the end of each flattened steak.

(continued)

Roll each steak from the mounded end and hold it in place with toothpicks. Turn the steaks seam side down.

Drizzle the steak rolls with olive oil and soy sauce.

Place the baking sheet at least 3 inches from the broiler flame to ensure that the toothpicks don't burn. Broil for 6 minutes, then turn the rolls and broil for an additional 7 minutes.

With a slotted spatula, remove the rolls to a serving platter, draining all excess liquid, and serve warm.

Mardi Gras Stew

PREP TIME: 25 minutes

COOK TIME: about 35 minutes

Our adaptation of a traditional dish that helps start the annual celebration off with a bang!

3 cups chicken stock (or our Classic Chicken Stock, page 66)

1/4 cup olive oil

2 teaspoons chopped onions

2 cloves garlic, pressed

1/2 cup chopped green bell peppers

1/2 cup chopped celery

1/2 cup sliced mushrooms

1/2 pound shrimp, raw, shelled and deveined

1/2 pound chicken breast halves, boneless and skinless, cut into 1-inch cubes

2 teaspoons paprika (hot or sweet)

1 teaspoon dried thyme

1/2 pound (about 6) sausage patties, fully cooked and crumbled (or our Freedom Sausage, page 23, fully cooked and crumbled)

1 teaspoon cayenne

1 teaspoon soy sauce

Additional hot sauce, as desired

2 teaspoons arrowroot powder dissolved in 4 teaspoons of water for thickening (optional)

In a very large soup pot or stockpot, over a low-medium flame, bring the stock to a simmer. Cover and keep at a very low simmer.

In a second very large soup pot, over a medium flame, warm the olive oil until hot (but not smoking). Add the onions and garlic and sauté until the onions begin to brown. Add the green peppers, celery, and mushrooms. Cook until the vegetables begin to soften (about 4 minutes), stirring often.

Add the shrimp, chicken cubes, paprika, and thyme. Stir to expose all surfaces to hot oil, and continue to cook for about 20 minutes, until the shrimp and chicken are thoroughly cooked (shrimp is opaque and chicken is opaque and white throughout).

Add the cooked sausage, cayenne, and soy sauce. Stir well. Remove from heat.

Raise heat under the stock to medium and remove the pot lid.

(continued)

Slowly add the shrimp and chicken mixture to the stock, ladle by ladle, allowing the stock to heat to a simmer between each addition. When the last ladle of mixture has been added, allow the mixture to reach a simmer, then remove from heat immediately.

Allow the stew to cool until all bubbling has stopped. If desired, for thickening, add the arrowroot mixture. Stir constantly to make certain the arrowroot mixture is distributed throughout.

Serve warm.

Jalapeño Nibblers

PREP TIME: 10 minutes
COOK TIME: 2 minutes

SERVINGS: 4
CARBS PER SERVING: 1 gram

We often start snacking on these as appetizers and never get to the rest of the meal.

Nonstick cooking spray
12 large mushroom caps (for stuffing)
12 pitted whole black ripe olives, drained and sliced

6 tablespoons crushed pork rinds
1/2 teaspoon black pepper
1/2 tablespoon dried basil
1/2 cup grated jalapeño cheese

Preheat the broiler.

Spray a baking sheet with nonstick cooking spray.

Invert the mushroom caps on the baking sheet so that they are not touching.

Line each mushroom cap with the slices of pitted black ripe olive.

In a blender, food processor, or by hand, crumble and combine the pork rinds, pepper, and basil.

Fill each mushroom cap with the pork rind mixture.

Top each mushroom cap with jalapeño cheese.

Transfer the baking sheet to the broiler and broil for 2 minutes, until the cheese is hot and bubbly, watching carefully to avoid burning.

Remove the mushroom caps from the broiler, transfer to a serving platter, and allow them to cool until a comfortable temperature for eating is reached.

Four-Spice Creamy Dip

PREP TIME: 3 minutes
COOK TIME: none

SERVINGS: 4 (¼ cup each)
CARBS PER SERVING: 4 grams

This combination of horseradish and bacon infused with blended spices adds lots of flavor to any salad, crudités, or steamed vegetables. We also love this dip with meat, fowl, or seafood.

1 cup creamed cottage cheese
2 tablespoons light whipping cream
1 tablespoon white prepared horseradish
½ teaspoon ground white pepper

Chili oil or hot sauce, as desired
½ teaspoon Hungarian (hot) paprika
4 slices bacon, cooked crisp and crumbled

Combine all the ingredients in a food processor, blender, or mixer and beat until smooth.

Cover and keep refrigerated until ready to use.

TANGY TEMPTATIONS

Dijon Stuffed Peppers

PREP TIME: 11 minutes
COOK TIME: none

SERVINGS: 2
CARBS PER SERVING: 3 grams

We discovered this easy no-cook meal on Grand Cayman Island. The restaurant lunches we were being served left us feeling too full to go snorkeling or diving for the rest of the day. So instead of going to the restaurant, we raided the nearby convenience store and grabbed everything that looked low-carb, although we had no idea how it would all work together. We liked the results so much, we made this dish three days running: a perfect summer lunch when you're on the go.

1 can (7½ ounces) red salmon with liquid (bones and skin removed)
½ cup minced celery
2 tablespoons white prepared horseradish
1 teaspoon Dijon mustard
½ teaspoon minced onion

1 teaspoon dried basil
3 ounces cream cheese, quartered
6 pitted green olives, drained and sliced
2 green bell peppers, left whole, cored and seeded from the top

In the bowl of an electric mixer at slow speed, combine the salmon and liquid from the can, celery, horseradish, mustard, onion, and basil. (Lots of hand mixing with a fork will do as well.)

Add the cream cheese chunks, one at a time, mixing well after each addition. Put aside.

Add the olive slices, reserving a few slices for garnish.

Fill the green peppers with the salmon mixture and garnish with the remaining olive slices.

Serve immediately or chill for 1 hour and serve cold.

Great with our Tofu Crisps (page 103).

Not Your Ordinary Burgers

PREP TIME: 6 minutes
COOK TIME: 15 to 25 minutes

SERVINGS: 6 (1 patty each)
CARBS PER SERVING: 2 grams

The cilantro and citrus juice, in combination, give these hamburgers a special zing. The three different proteins deliver a not-your-ordinary-burger flavor.

1/2 pound ground beef (sirloin, rib eye, or cut of your choice)
1/2 pound ground turkey
1/2 pound ground pork
1/2 cup crushed pork rinds (optional)

2 eggs, beaten
1/2 cup chopped cilantro
4 cloves garlic, minced
1/4 cup chopped scallions
1/4 cup lemon or lime juice
Salt, pepper, and cayenne, as desired

Combine all the ingredients in a large bowl. Mix thoroughly with your hands so that all the ingredients are equally distributed. Divide into six patties of equal size.

Fry the patties in olive oil, broil them, or grill them until thoroughly cooked.

These burgers are great with one of our three homemade hot sauces (pages 259, 260, and 261) or topped with a slice of jalapeño cheese.

Kanya's Cabbage

PREP TIME: 8 minutes
COOK TIME: 5 minutes

SERVINGS: 4
CARBS PER SERVING: 2 grams

A young woman who had recently started volunteering at the homeless shelter where we helped out brought this dish to the annual Thanksgiving dinner. We loved it and so did the shelter residents, but some of the other volunteers ridiculed her behind her back for bringing what they assumed was a "cheap" contribution. Weeks later, we all discovered that, just off the streets herself, she had gone without food for two days in order to afford the ingredients for this dish from her homeland.

1   fresh red or green chili
    pepper*
6   cups thinly sliced green
    cabbage
1/2 teaspoon ground ginger
1/8 teaspoon ground cumin
1/4 teaspoon dried oregano

1/8 teaspoon dried basil
1   clove garlic, crushed
1/4 teaspoon salt
2   cups sour cream
1/4 cup grated Parmesan or
    Romano cheese

Wearing gloves, core, seed, and quarter the chili pepper.

In a large soup pot over a high flame, bring 4 cups of water to a boil.

Remove the soup pot from the heat and carefully add the chili pepper quarters, sliced cabbage, ginger, cumin, oregano, basil, garlic, and salt.

Cover the pot and return it to the heat, bringing the cabbage mixture to a boil. Allow the mixture to boil for 3 minutes.

Immediately remove the pot from the heat and drain the cabbage in a colander. Discard liquid.

Wearing gloves, carefully remove the chili pepper quarters and discard.

*NOTE: When handling chili peppers, it's always a good idea to wear rubber or latex gloves. The pepper can burn and irritate your hands even if you are not aware of any tiny cuts or abrasions that may exist. Be certain not to touch your face or eyes or any other area that may be vulnerable to damage or irritation. Immediately wash knife, cutting surfaces, and gloves when finished.

(continued)

Transfer the mixture to a large serving bowl, add the sour cream, and toss well.

Top with Parmesan or Romano cheese and serve warm.

Tangy Fried Chicken

PREP TIME: 6 minutes
COOK TIME: 16 minutes

SERVINGS: 4
CARBS PER SERVING: 4 grams

We thought that we had invented this recipe until our friend, Kim, informed us that it was an old Vietnamese dish. "With Parmesan and sour cream?" we asked incredulously. "Yes," she assured us. We still don't believe her.

2   cups sour cream
1/2 teaspoon ground ginger
2   cloves garlic, minced (or
    1 teaspoon garlic powder)
1/2 teaspoon dried rosemary
    Salt and pepper, as desired

1   pound chicken breast
    halves, boneless and
    skinless, about 1/2 inch
    thick, divided into
    4 pieces
1   cup grated Parmesan or
    Romano cheese
1/4 cup olive oil

In a bowl combine the sour cream, ginger, garlic, and rosemary. Mix well.

Add salt and pepper as desired. Add the chicken and mix well to cover.

Cover the bowl and place it in the refrigerator to marinate for 2 hours.

Transfer the grated cheese to a plate.

Heat the olive oil in a large skillet over a medium flame to warm (but not smoking).

Remove the chicken pieces from the marinade, discarding the marinade.

Dip each chicken section in the grated cheese to coat both sides. Transfer the chicken to the hot oil (carefully, as it will splatter).

Cook on one side until deep golden brown (about 8 minutes), then turn with a spatula, careful to maintain coating. Cook until the other side is the same deep golden brown and thoroughly cooked (another 8 minutes).

Serve warm.

Tapenade with a Twist

PREP TIME: 6 minutes
COOK TIME: none

SERVINGS: 4
CARBS PER SERVING: 2 grams

Tapenades are classic Mediterranean spreads made from black (preferably Kalamata) olives. Recently, they have become popular in this country and for good reason: they're low-carb, easy to make, and absolutely delicious. Once you've tried this basic recipe, you might want to personalize it by adding your favorite low-carb ingredients.

1 clove garlic, crushed
1 cup Kalamata olives, pitted and drained
1/4 cup orange zest
1 teaspoon lime juice

5 anchovies, drained and mashed
2 tablespoons olive oil
1 hard-boiled egg, shelled and quartered

Combine all ingredients in a food processor and process until the mixture forms a paste. Makes about 1 cup.

Transfer the tapenade to a covered dish and refrigerate for at least two hours.

Serve with our Tofu Crisps (page 103), as stuffing for celery stalks, or as a thick dip for green pepper wedges. Wonderful when spread on a slice of mozzarella cheese!

Christmas Pot Roast

PREP TIME: 15 minutes
COOK TIME: 3 hours

SERVINGS: 8
CARBS PER SERVING: 3 grams

We like to make extra meat dishes around Christmas. With all of the extra carbs that holiday visitors bring, it's a lifesaver to be able to reach into the refrigerator and pull out a treat that's absolutely delicious and still low-carb. This is our old standby. We can always count on it to get us through the holidays without feeling deprived.

2 pounds beef chuck roast	1/2 teaspoon salt
2 tablespoons dry red wine	2 tablespoons butter
2 tablespoons white vinegar	2 cups sliced mushrooms
2 tablespoons soy sauce	2 stalks celery, trimmed and
2 bay leaves	minced
1 teaspoon dry mustard	1/4 cup capers
1/2 teaspoon ground black pepper	

Place the roast in the bottom of a deep roasting pan with a cover. Set it aside.

In a small bowl combine the wine, vinegar, soy sauce, bay leaves, mustard, black pepper, and salt. Add 1 cup of water and stir well. Transfer the mixture to the bottom of the roasting pan.

Add enough additional water to the roasting pan to completely cover the meat with 1 inch of water. Cover the pan and refrigerate overnight.

To cook, pour off the marinade until half of the meat can be seen above the marinade line. Place an oven thermometer in the thickest portion of the roast, away from any bone.

Preheat the oven to 325°F.

Cover the pan and roast for about 3 hours, basting several times.

One hour prior to removing the roast from the oven, heat the butter in a small saucepan over a low flame. Sauté the mushrooms, celery, and capers until the mushrooms are golden brown. Add the vegetable mixture and cooking liquid to the roasting pan. Baste several times during the last hour of roasting.

(continued)

Remove the pan from the oven when the thermometer indicates that the roast is well done.

Remove the bay leaves. Using a slotted spoon, transfer the vegetables from the gravy in the bottom of the pan to a separate serving dish.

Transfer the meat to a carving board, slice it, and serve it hot with au jus gravy. Refrigerate the leftovers for lots of good low-carb snacks.

Quick and Tangy
Mushroom Curry

PREP TIME: 9 minutes	**SERVINGS:** 4
COOK TIME: 10 to 11 minutes	**CARBS PER SERVING:** 3 grams

You're on a luxury dive boat, two hours outside of Cairns, Australia, just entering the Great Barrier Reef. The best snorkeling and diving in the world awaits you and . . . darn, they had to go and serve that awesome mushroom curry again. Now you've got to make the hardest decision of the day: eat or snorkel. Oh, well. The Great Barrier Reef will have to wait.

2 tablespoons butter
3 tablespoons olive oil
2 tablespoons chopped onions
1 teaspoon curry powder
1/4 teaspoon ground cinnamon
1/2 teaspoon salt
2 cups sliced mushrooms

2 tablespoons chopped tomato
1/4 cup heavy whipping cream
Ground black pepper and/or cayenne, as desired
1/2 cup grated cheese (cheddar, American, Swiss, or Monterey Jack)

Heat the butter and olive oil in a medium-size saucepan over a medium flame. Sauté the onions, stirring often, until the onions turn translucent, then golden brown (3 to 4 minutes).

Add the curry powder, cinnamon, and salt and cook for 1 additional minute, stirring often.

Add the mushrooms and tomato. Stir to combine well.

Cook, stirring often, until the mushrooms turn golden and are soft (about 3 minutes). Remove from heat.

Reduce heat to low, add the cream to the saucepan, stir well, and return the saucepan to the heat. Stir and warm the cream but do not boil (about 3 minutes).

Remove from heat, season as desired, stir, divide into two portions, and top with grated cheese.

Serve warm.

Citrus Flounder

PREP TIME: 5 minutes
COOK TIME: 15 to 20 minutes

SERVINGS: 4
CARBS PER SERVING: 4 grams

We were having four guests for dinner. Two didn't eat beef or pork, one didn't eat chicken, and the fourth didn't like fish. Along with this recipe, we served a beef dish, but our non-fish-eater never got to it. "It doesn't have that fishy taste," he proclaimed, finishing off his second serving. We took that as high praise.

3 tablespoons olive oil
1/4 cup finely chopped green bell pepper
1/2 cup chopped celery
2 tablespoons chopped onion
1 tablespoon chopped fresh dill
1 tablespoon chopped fresh parsley
1/2 teaspoon ground ginger

1 1/2 teaspoons lemon zest
1 teaspoon lime zest
2 tablespoons lime juice
1 teaspoon soy sauce (optional)
Salt and ground white pepper, as desired
4 flounder fillets (4 to 6 ounces each), completely deboned

Preheat the oven to 350°F.

Lightly grease a baking dish with 1 tablespoon of the olive oil. Set aside.

Warm the remaining olive oil in a medium-size saucepan over a medium flame and sauté the green pepper, celery, and onion, stirring often, until the onion begins to turn brown around the edges and the celery and green peppers soften (about 7 minutes),

Add the dill, parsley, and ginger. Mix well to coat and then remove from heat.

Add the lemon zest, lime zest, lime juice, and soy sauce. Mix well. Season with salt and white pepper as desired.

Place the flounder fillets in the baking dish. Spread 1/4 of the vegetable mixture on each fillet.

Bake for 7 to 10 minutes, or until the fish is opaque and flakes with a fork.

Zesty Clam Cups

| PREP TIME: 8 minutes | SERVINGS: 4 |
| COOK TIME: 2 minutes | CARBS PER SERVING: 2 grams |

The blend of flavors in this dish may surprise you. It's deep and rich, smoky and tangy and refreshing—all at the same time. The lime zest adds a perfect balance (lemon zest will do, too!). When we're in a rush, we don't bother broiling the mushroom caps; we just stuff them, grab them, and go.

Nonstick cooking spray
2 cans (6 to 8 ounces each) ready-to-eat, minced clams, drained
1 cup sour cream
1/2 teaspoon pressed garlic
1/4 cup crushed pork rinds (or 2 slices bacon, cooked crisp and crumbled)
12 large mushroom caps (for stuffing)
1 tablespoon lime zest

Preheat the broiler.

Spray a baking sheet with nonstick cooking spray. Set aside.

In a large bowl, combine the clams, sour cream, garlic, and pork rinds. Mix well. Set aside.

Invert the mushroom caps on a baking sheet so that they are not touching. Fill each mushroom cap with the clam and sour cream mixture.

Place the baking sheet under the broiler and broil for 2 minutes, until filling is warmed, watching carefully to avoid burning.

Remove the baking sheet from the broiler and allow the mushrooms to rest until they're cool enough to eat.

Top each mushroom with lime zest, for garnish as well as for a balance of flavors.

Easter Lamb

PREP TIME: 10 minutes

COOK TIME: approximately 1¼ hours

SERVINGS: 8

CARBS PER SERVING: 0 grams

The bus from Mt. Surprise, Northern Queensland (population: 65), to the city of Cairns ran only three times a week, when it was running at all, and at the start of Easter vacation, it wasn't. The bus had broken down and it looked like we were going to be stranded at the combination post office/gas station/ticket office/grocery store/only-lunch-counter-in-town, sleeping on the bench outside and eating Vegemite on white bread for the next three days. Then the woman at the lunch counter surprised us by offering two portions of her own homemade Easter dinner lamb. Afterward, she connected us up with the limping bus and got us back to the city in time to continue our holiday. Here's our version of the lamb dish she shared.

1 3-pound loin of lamb roast	1 teaspoon dried basil
½ cup chopped fresh mint leaves	½ teaspoon ground ginger
2 tablespoons soy sauce	1 teaspoon dried thyme
2 teaspoons lemon juice	1 teaspoon dried sage
3 cloves garlic, crushed	2 tablespoons olive oil
	Salt and pepper, as desired

Preheat the oven to 375°F. Place the lamb, fat side up, on a rack in a roasting pan with 1½ inches of water below the rack. Maintain at least 1 inch of water throughout cooking.

In a small bowl combine the remaining ingredients. Mix thoroughly.

Make small slits on the surface of the lamb and rub part of the mixture into the slits well. Rub the remainder of the mixture over the surface of the lamb.

Insert a meat thermometer into the thickest part of the meat, away from any bone. Place the lamb in the oven. After 15 minutes, reduce the heat to 325°F. Roast for 1 hour or until the internal temperature reaches at least 170°F.

Remove the pan from the oven and allow the roast to sit for 10 minutes before slicing. Serve warm with au jus gravy.

(continued)

This meat is also delicious served cold with our Instant Onion Dip (page 225) or topped with mustard and wrapped in a lettuce or spinach leaf.

Luscious Chicken Leftovers

PREP TIME: 5 minutes
COOK TIME: 26 minutes

SERVINGS: 2
CARBS PER SERVING: 2 grams

Leftovers spur the most creative recipes. Instead of grabbing a slab of cold chicken, take a few minutes to make a gourmet treat.

1/2 head green cabbage
2 tablespoons butter
1 cup sliced mushrooms
1/2 teaspoon ground ginger
1 teaspoon paprika (hot or sweet)
2 teaspoons dried basil

1 cup sour cream
1/2 cup grated Swiss cheese
1/4 cup chopped fresh parsley
2 leftover chicken breast halves, fully cooked
Salt and pepper, as desired
Lemon and lime wedges

Preheat the oven to 350°F.

Cut the cabbage in half.

Place 1 inch of water in a deep skillet, add the cabbage, and turn the heat to high. Cover and heat for 3 minutes. Turn off the heat, pour off the water, and keep the skillet covered. Set aside.

In a small saucepan over a low flame, melt the butter until foamy but not brown. Add the mushrooms, ginger, paprika, and basil. Stir well and cook until the mushrooms start to turn golden (about 3 minutes). Add the sour cream, cheese, and parsley. Stir until the cheese is melted.

Lightly grease a shallow baking pan (at least 1 inch high). Center the cooked chicken breasts and cabbage in the pan and top with the sour cream sauce.

Sprinkle with parsley, add salt and pepper as desired, and bake for 20 minutes.

Remove and serve warm. Drizzle with fresh lemon and lime juice.

Chicken Vindaloo

PREP TIME: 10 minutes
COOK TIME: 40 minutes

SERVINGS: 4
CARBS PER SERVING: 1 gram

Don't be daunted by the long list of ingredients in this recipe. Once you assemble them, it's easy going from there. Although the spices work well together, if you don't have one or two or want to add a few of your own, feel free to be creative. This is a different dish every time we make it.

4 tablespoons olive oil
2 teaspoons chopped onion
4 cloves garlic, peeled
1 section (1 inch) fresh ginger root
1 tablespoon cumin seeds
1 tablespoon coriander seeds
1 teaspoon ground turmeric
1/2 teaspoon ground black pepper
Salt, as desired
1/4 cup white vinegar
1/4 teaspoon ground cardamom
Dried hot red chili peppers*, as desired
1 stick cinnamon
1 pound chicken breast halves, cut into 1-inch cubes
2 teaspoons finely crushed tomato
2 cups chicken stock (or our Classic Chicken Stock, page 66) or water

Heat 1 tablespoon of the olive oil in a small skillet over a low-medium flame until hot (but not smoking). Add the onions and sauté, stirring often, until the onion turns golden brown. Remove the onions from the pan and drain on a paper towel.

To make the vindaloo paste, place the browned onions, garlic, ginger, cumin seeds, coriander seeds, turmeric, pepper, salt as desired, and vinegar in a blender and purée until smooth. Add a teaspoon or two of the olive oil as needed for processing.

Add the cardamom and chili peppers. Grate 1/4 teaspoon of the

*NOTE: When handling chili peppers, it's always a good idea to wear rubber or latex gloves. The pepper can burn and irritate your hands even if you are not aware of any tiny cuts or abrasions that may exist. Be certain not to touch your face or eyes or any other area that may be vulnerable to damage or irritation. Immediately wash knife, cutting surfaces, and gloves when finished.

(continued)

fresh cinnamon and add to the blender. Purée the mixture once again until smooth. Set aside.

Heat the remaining olive oil in a large skillet over a medium-high flame. Add the chicken cubes, stirring continuously so that all sides are browned (about 5 minutes).

Add the vindaloo paste and stir so the chicken is coated on all sides. Continue to cook for an additional 5 minutes, stirring often.

Add the crushed tomato and 1 cup of the chicken stock or water, a bit at a time, stirring after each addition.

Bring to a boil, then lower the heat, uncovered, and simmer gently for 30 minutes, or until the chicken is tender and thoroughly cooked.

The finished chicken should be coated with the thick sauce. Replace the chicken stock or water as needed during cooking to keep the chicken from drying out. To thicken the sauce, uncover the chicken and simmer at a rolling boil. Stir often to prevent sticking and ensure even coverage of sauce.

Serve the chicken warm over shredded raw cabbage or with cool cucumber slices.

Wilted Spinach–Bacon Salad

PREP TIME: 10 minutes
COOK TIME: 5 minutes

SERVINGS: 4
CARBS PER SERVING: 2 grams

We first discovered the salad that inspired this dish in the old Russian Tea Room next to Carnegie Hall. The waiter said it was rumored to be Leo Tolstoy's favorite and one that was "both satisfying and light, feeding his creative genius." We believed him . . . until we remembered that Tolstoy was a vegetarian.

8 slices raw bacon, cut into 1-inch pieces
3 tablespoons olive oil
1 cup drained sauerkraut
12 ripe black olives, drained and sliced

1/2 pound fresh spinach, trimmed, washed, and dried
2 hard-boiled eggs, shelled and quartered
   Alfalfa sprouts (optional)

Cook the bacon in a large skillet over a medium flame, until crisp. Turn heat to low. Remove the pan from the heat and transfer the bacon to a dry plate. Retain 3 tablespoons of drippings in the pan.

Before returning the pan to low heat, add to the pan drippings the olive oil, sauerkraut, and olive slices, in that order. Be careful of splatter. Stir.

Heat the mixture for 2 minutes over a low flame, stirring constantly. Turn off heat.

Add half of the spinach to the skillet. Toss to coat the leaves well. Do not cook.

Use a slotted spoon to transfer the contents of the skillet into a large salad bowl, allowing excess oil mixture to drip back into the skillet.

Sprinkle the spinach in the bowl with half of the bacon, crumbling the bacon as you add it.

Add the remaining spinach to the skillet, toss to coat the leaves with oil, and then add to the rest of the ingredients in the bowl.

Toss the entire salad and top with hard-boiled egg quarters, alfalfa sprouts, and the remaining bacon, crumbled.

Serve warm.

INDEX

in Crunchy Vegetable-Beef Soup,
115–16
in Curried Okra with Gingered
"Rice, 140–41
in Daintree Marinade, 91–92
in Damyanti's Curried Salad, 132
in Grab-and-Go Low-Carb Sushi,
195–96
in Grits, Sausage, and Gravy, 161
in Kung Bao Chicken, 60
in Low-Carb Macaroni and Cheese,
65
in Mashed "Potatoes," 210
in Nearly Fried Rice, 56
in Nearly Nine Dragons Lemon
Shrimp, 49
in Perfect Low-Carb Potato Salad, 18
in Tuscan Marinade, 174
cheddar cheese
in Cheese Pop 'Ems, 229
in Edmonton Pork and Beans, 149
in Grab-and-Go BBQ, 21
in Olive Cheese Spread, 243
cheese
in Almost Potatoes Au Gratin, 148
in Anytime Antipasto, 175
Cheese Pop 'Ems, 229
Cheese Sauce, 253–54
in Chicken Salad Anise, 133
Chicken with Green Cheese, 147
Chili Beef and Cheese, 157–58
in Classic Pesto, 178
in Classic Tofu Burgers, 205–6
Crisp & Crackly Cheese Crackers,
104
in Friday Night "Steak," 218
in Harvard Mushroom Morsels, 90
in Hearty Meatless Casserole,
214–15
Hot Spinach Cheese Dip, 73
Left Bank Boursin, 242
in Lemon Zest Chicken Salad, 98
Low-Carb Macaroni and Cheese, 65
in Luscious Chicken Leftovers, 290
in North Queensland Greek Salad,
109
Olive Cheese Spread, 243
in Piccadilly Circus Sirloin Steaks,
125–26

in Pizza Crisps, 168
Porcupine Cheese Ball, 93
in Quick & Tangy Mushroom Curry,
285
Rapid Roquefort Cheese Sauce for
Leftovers, 237
in Seafood Dijon Cobb Salad, 233
in Timeless Quiche, 71
in Tofu Western Melt, 212
in Waldorf Lamb Salad, 105
See also Brie; cheddar cheese; cottage
cheese; cream cheese; mozzarella
cheese; Parmesan cheese; ricotta
cheese
Cheese-Filled Treats, 25–43
Almost No-Carb Parmesan Puffs, 27
Canadian Cheese Soup, 38
Chewy Cheese Mozzarella Logs, 32
Chicken Provençal, 40–41
Four-Cheese Veggie Stuffer, 42
Green Pepper with Cheese Dip, 39
Midnight Pizza, 35–36
Mushroom-Brie Omelet, 43
No Worries Caesar Salad, 28
Quick Carbonara, 31
Savory Tarts, 34
Silky-Smooth Cheese Sauce, 33
Velvety Cheese Soufflé, 37
Winter Night Tuna Melt, 29–30
Cheesy and Smooth Crabmeat
Casserole, 253–54
Cheesy Creamed Spinach, 245
Chewy Cheese Mozzarella Logs, 32
Chia Pets, Tuna, 170–71
Chiba Pork Roast, 189–90
chicken
Asian Chicken Nuggets, 194
in Cajun Grill, 11
Chicken Medallions, 107
Chicken Parmesan Romana, 173
Chicken Pavarotti, 167
Chicken Provençal, 40–41
Chicken Salad Anise, 133
Chicken Vindaloo, 291–92
Chicken with Green Cheese, 147
Chill-Fighting Chicken Fricassee, 79
Chinese Chicken/Beef Stock, 66–67
Classic Chicken Stock, 66–67
in Classic Chop Suey, 54

French Brussels Sprouts, 129
Friday Night "Steak," 218
Fried Rice, Nearly, 56
Fried Steak, Crystal River, 120
Fujian Duck, 52
Fundamental Fish Stock, 185

Gansu Pulled Pork, 47–48
Gentle Asparagus Purée, 70
Ginger Cream Shrimp, 128
Gingered "Rice," Curried Okra,
 140–41
glutamates, unwanted additions, 4–6
Grab-and-Go BBQ, 21
Grab-and-Go Low-Carb Sushi, 195–96
Gratin, Almost Potatoes Au, 148
Gravy, Grits, and Sausage, 161
Great American Cookout Pork Roast,
 78
Greek Salad, North Queensland, 109
green beans
 in Canadian Logger Stew, 155–56
 in Edmonton Pork and Beans, 149
 in Hearty Meatless Casserole,
  214–15
 in Quick Carbonara, 31
 in Yellow Dragon Tofu, 198
green bell peppers
 in Chicken Pavarotti, 167
 in Chili Beef and Cheese, 157–58
 in Classic Tofu Burgers, 205–6
 in Cool Green Pinwheel Salad, 85
 in Daikon Salad, 192
 Dijon Stuffed Peppers, 277
 in Fast Foo Young, 226
 Green Pepper with Cheese Dip, 39
 in Green Salsa, 97
 Kiwi Green Pepper Steak, 55
 in Mardi Gras Stew, 270–71
 in North Queensland Greek Salad,
  109
 in Old-Fashioned "Chicken"
  Casserole, 216
 in On-the-Run Tuna Salad Cups, 232
 in Piccadilly Circus Sirloin Steaks,
  125–26
 in Pizza Crisps, 168
 Roasted Green Pepper Sauce, 162
 in Salmon Scones, 163

 in Scaloppine Palermo, 179
 in Shrimp and Bacon Bowl, 112–13
 in Smooth and Cheesy Crabmeat
  Casserole, 253–54
 in Spicy (or Mild) Vegetarian Stir-Fry,
  209
 in Sunday Dinner Roast Chicken,
  159–60
 in Tuscan Marinade, 174
Green Salsa, 97
Grill, Cajun, 11
Grits, Sausage, and Gravy, 161

Harvard Mushroom Morsels, 90
Hawaiian Hot-Hot Sauce, 261
healthy selfishness, 2, 3
Hearty Feasts, 145–63
 Almost Potatoes Au Gratin, 148
 Canadian Logger Stew, 155–56
 Chicken with Green Cheese, 147
 Chili Beef and Cheese, 157–58
 Crock-Pot Tender Roast Beef, 153
 Edmonton Pork and Beans, 149
 Grits, Sausage, and Gravy, 161
 Herb-Encrusted Steak, 150
 Independence Day Flounder, 151–52
 Roasted Green Pepper Sauce, 162
 Salmon Scones, 163
 Sunday Dinner Roast Chicken,
  159–60
 Tasty Turkey Burgers, 154
Hearty Meatless Casserole, 214–15
Heller, Rachael F., Richard F., 6, 29
Herb Blend Southern Crusty Coating,
 119
Herb-Encrusted Steak, 150
Homemade Hot Sauce, 259
Hot and Puffy Lamb Chops, 263
Hot and Sour Mushrooms, Osaka,
 200–201
Hot and Sour Soup, Silk Road, 57–58
Hot-Hot Sauce, Hawaiian, 261
Hot Sauce, Homemade, 259
Hot Spinach Cheese Dip, 73
Hungarian Creamed Mushrooms, 72

Independence Day Flounder, 151–52
ingredients, 3–4
Instant Onion Dip, 225